# The Elusive Orgasm

"Filled with practical advice and sound suggestions, *The Elusive Orgasm* is sure to help women overcome the inhibitions or interferences that are preventing them from enjoying orgasmic pleasure. Written with the understanding and knowledge that only an experienced sex therapist can offer, Dr. Cass has produced a book that will prove incredibly helpful to scores of women. I recommend it highly!"
—SANDRA LEIBLUM, PhD, Director,
Center of Sexual and Relationship Health, UMDNJ—Robert
Wood Johnson Medical School, author of *Getting the Sex You Want*

"An outstandingly readable book, with excellent illustrations. In a thoroughly modern way Dr. Cass provides her readers with invaluable information and advice. Such knowledge enhances the lives of women *and* their sexual partners. Mothers read this book and then pass it on to your daughters!"
—ROSEMARY COATES, PhD,
Sexology Programs, School of Public Health,
Curtin University, Australia

"*The Elusive Orgasm* is an important book for all women, their partners and health professionals. It takes a woman by the hand and gently guides her to sexual satisfaction and pleasure. What fun to read!"
—BEVERLY WHIPPLE, PhD, RN,
vice president, World Association
for Sexology, coauthor, *The G-Spot*

"[A] sexual bible."
—*OUT* magazine

"[R]eminds us that orgasms are not essential to good or even great sex. . . . A very helpful and reassuring book that is more than a guide to having orgasms, it is a book about having good sex. Clinicians who treat women with arousal and orgasm difficulties will find *The Elusive Orgasm* an extremely helpful adjunct to therapy."
—*Journal of Sex and Marital Therapy*

# The Elusive Orgasm

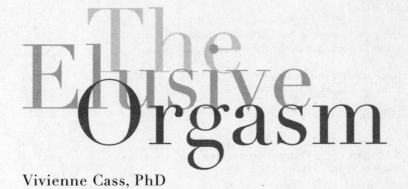

# The Elusive Orgasm

Vivienne Cass, PhD

a woman's guide to why she can't
and how she can orgasm

Da Capo

LIFE
LONG

A Member of the Perseus Books Group

Copyright © 2007 by Vivienne Cass, PhD
Illustrations by Medical Arts
First published in Australia by Brightfire Press in 2004. This edition published by arrangement.

Designed by Pauline Neuwirth, Neuwirth & Associates, Inc.
Set in 11 point Bembo by the Perseus Books Group

Cataloging-in-Publication data for this book is available from the Library of Congress.

ISBN: 978-1-60094-023-1

Published by Da Capo Press
A Member of the Perseus Books Group
www.dacapopress.com

Note: The information in this book is true and complete to the best of our knowledge. This book is intended only as an informative guide for those wishing to know more about health issues. In no way is this book intended to replace, countermand, or conflict with the advice given to you by your own physician. The ultimate decision concerning care should be made between you and your doctor. We strongly recommend you follow his or her advice. Information in this book is general and is offered with no guarantees on the part of the authors or Da Capo Press. The authors and publisher disclaim all liability in connection with the use of this book. The names and identifying details of people associated with events described in this book have been changed. Any similarity to actual persons is coincidental.

Da Capo Press books are available at special discounts for bulk purchases in the U.S. by corporations, institutions, and other organizations. For more information, please contact the Special Markets Department at the Perseus Books Group, 2300 Chestnut Street, Suite 200, Philadelphia, PA, 19103, or call (800) 810-4145, ext. 5000, or e-mail special.markets@perseusbooks.com.

10 9 8 7 6 5

*This book is dedicated to my mother,*
*who has always encouraged and supported my endeavors.*

# contents

# illustrations

# acknowledgments

MY HEARTFELT THANKS to the following people, whose skills and support have been greatly appreciated:

Dr. Gwen Leavesley, women's sexual health specialist and previously director of the Family Planning Association in Western Australia, who unreservedly drew upon her considerable experience and knowledge in women's sexual health to review the sections related to sexual medicine and to answer my numerous phone calls, which usually started with, "Gwen, have you got a minute. . . . ?" (when I really meant, "Have you got much more than a minute. . . . ?")

Dr. Levent Efe, medical illustrator, who created the innovative and excellent illustrations, enthusiastically responding to my request that they be helpful to all women regardless of background and levels of education, and patiently attending to my need for everything to be "just right."

Dr. Helen O'Connell, foremost researcher of the clitoral anatomy, who made time in her busy schedule to check the illustrations against her firsthand knowledge of women's genital anatomy.

Dr. Shona Penhale, the young American medical researcher studying the nerve networks to the clitoris, who willingly shared her research findings with me.

Catherine Hammond, a sharp-eyed editor, who helped shape the manuscript into something I could be proud of, and who gave me support and encouragement well beyond her official role.

Renée Sedliar, editor at Marlowe & Company, who managed, via e-mails, to convey a respect and confidence in my work. My respect and confidence in *her* are returned in kind.

Lesley and Michael Tunnecliffe from Bayside Books, Jackie Aitken and Lea Smith from WA Book Agencies, and fellow psychologist and bookseller Zish Zimbinski from Mosaic Books for their support and willingness to share valuable knowledge.

Virginia Hailes and Ruth Wykes who, despite dire warnings about the thankless job of proofreading, happily took up the challenge anyway . . . thank goodness!

And to my family and special friends, especially Debbie, Susan, Robyn, Joan, Anne, Gerty, Margaret, Chris, Di, Clive, Eva, Audrey, Sol, and Shelley, for continuing to ask, "How's the book going?" and then patiently listening as I gave them yet another step-by-step account.

# introduction:
## the elusive author

I THINK IT'S only fair that you know something about me. After all, discussing orgasms is not the same as talking about what to cook for dinner. Wouldn't it be nice if it were that simple? Unfortunately, few of us live in societies where sex is accepted so positively.

So, let me begin with the serious stuff. I started out as a bookkeeper, then public servant, then teacher, before becoming a clinical psychologist and psychotherapist. I became professionally involved in the sexuality area at a time when such a thing was considered a sure sign of secret nymphomania (an obsession with sex).

Somehow I survived and have been in private practice now for nearly thirty years (although I can't imagine where the time's gone). I've worked mostly with adults, covering all sorts of psychological difficulties, as well as sexual issues.

Since the 1970s I've taught courses on sexual therapy at universities and to health professionals and given talks and lectures on sexuality and psychology to community groups, professionals, and the general public. I also give my fair share of media interviews, since (as we all know) sexuality and human relations are favorite topics with journalists and conference organizers.

Also of interest to me is the area of sexual orientation. In 1979 I published the first of over a dozen papers and book chapters on the way people develop the identities of "homosexual," "gay," "lesbian," and "bisexual." Happily, my ideas are still being used by therapists and researchers even today.

In the mid-1980s I was asked to set up counseling services in the area of HIV/AIDS and, as a result of my experiences, published a book, *There's More to Sex Than AIDS: The A to Z Guide to Safe Sex*.

So, that's it in a nutshell. No stunning overnight career as an Internet millionaire. No worldwide exposure as a $10,000-a-day model. No one beating a path to my door to play TV host. Oh, wait . . . I did have a yearlong stint as one-half of a duo, singing and playing guitar at a local hotel (until it was sold and our services "no-longer-required-thank-you"). And I did have a few moments of fame co-hosting a weekly radio program, *You're Only Human*, for two years. It was about the way humans imitate animals. Just kidding!

For those of you who must know the star sign of an author before you read their books, I was born under the sign of Capricorn—and yes, I'm too serious, much too practical, and I have a tendency to focus on my work instead of those around me. Fortunately, I enjoy music and balance out the serious stuff with raucous renditions of "Climb Every Mountain" (which, as you'll find out in chapter 3, is required singing for any sexual therapist).

Well, that about sums it up. Oh, yes . . . I'm told I belong to the baby boomers, but there's nothing too babylike about me these days—and I certainly don't "boom" much any more.

$$\backsim$$

P.S.: WRITING A book is damn hard. Everyone knows this. So why haven't I learned my lesson and turned to gardening instead?

Well, if you must know, it started with my concern for the many women who live in remote country areas and don't have access to psychological help, especially in the area of sexual therapy.

And then I thought about the women who are too embarrassed or shy to make an appointment to see a sexual therapist, even if one *is* available.

And then I pondered over what to do with thirty-odd years of therapy experience when I retire.

So, you see, in no time I'd talked myself into writing *The Elusive Orgasm*. And the thought that I might be able to cheer up someone having difficulties with orgasm dangled like a carrot in front of me and kept me going—even when the thought of typing the word "orgasm" yet again made me want to scream. (Okay, so now you also know I'm not the calmest person in the world!)

◎

ANOTHER P.S.: THIS is probably a good time to let you know that, despite my peculiarities, the following organizations are still happy to have me as a member:

- The Society for the Scientific Study of Sexuality (USA)
- The New York Academy of Science (USA)
- The International Society for the Study of Women's Sexual Health
- Editorial Board, *Journal of Homosexuality* (USA)
- Australian Society of Sex Educators, Researchers and Therapists (AUS)
- Western Australian Sexology Society (AUS)
- Australian Psychological Society (AUS)
- Independently Practising Clinical Psychologists Association (AUS)
- Australian Society of Authors (AUS)

# The Elusive Orgasm

# to begin with . . .

THERE ARE SOME women who do not orgasm during sex and are quite content with this. Then again, there are some women who are extremely dissatisfied with this situation. Strange, don't you think, how something that's acceptable to one woman is seen as a problem by another? Yet, women differ in other areas, so why not in the way they express their sexuality?

This book has been written for any woman who finds it difficult to orgasm *and is not content with this situation.* So, if you do not orgasm *and are quite happy,* save yourself the cost of the book—you don't have a problem (even if someone else tries to tell you otherwise). Of course, you may be interested in learning a little more about women's orgasm and buy the book for this reason. Hopefully, your curiosity will be met.

Did you know that a little baby girl, just a few months old, can have an orgasm by touching her clitoris or pressing her legs together and rocking gently? It's true! Of course, the baby has no understanding of what she's doing or feeling, and we could not call her experience "sexual," as we would for an adult. But she can experience a physical sensation that appears to be pleasurable and relaxing. And her vagina becomes wet, just as it does for an adult woman who is aroused.

I suppose you're now wondering,

---

But if this is so natural for babies, how come adult women—like me—are having problems with orgasm?

---

Exactly! What has happened to stop us using our natural ability to orgasm? This is the question I want to talk about in *The Elusive Orgasm*. The truth is, there are many adult women who have lost this ability.

One American survey found that in the twelve months prior to the study being carried out, *nearly one-third* of the women they investigated (31.6%) had never, rarely, or only sometimes felt an orgasm. And, *more than two-thirds* of women in the survey (71.4%) did not always orgasm during sex with a partner.[1]

Australian women are similar to American women with *nearly one-third* (28.6%) being unable to orgasm for a month or more in the previous twelve months.[2] In Europe, however, less women seem to have orgasm difficulties (4 to 10%).[3] Don't ask me why. It's still a bit of a mystery.

Do you think that having orgasms and being happy always go together? Think again. They don't! In the American survey, nearly half the women who *rarely, never, or sometimes had an orgasm* (48.1%) described themselves as *very happy*. And, of the women who had no orgasm difficulties, about *one-third* did *not* describe themselves as "very happy" (36%). Like I say, there's a lot more to being happy than having orgasms.

So what happened—from the moment you were born—that now stops you from climaxing or having an orgasm as easily as you'd like? I'm sure you've asked yourself this same question. But how easy has it been to find the answer? For many, not easy at all. You may not have access to a professional person with the right training. Books (not to mention bookshops) may not be available where you live. Perhaps you're too embarrassed to talk to anyone. You may have even tried different methods and found they didn't help.

So, I can understand if you're feeling a bit impatient or half-hearted.

---

Well, yes I am. But I've had my problem
for quite a while now, so I just want to get straight to
the point: how do I fix it?

---

Good question! We'll get to that soon enough. But first, you need to identify what kind of orgasm difficulty you have and why. This is important if you're going to choose the right program to overcome it.

You need to first *understand* your orgasm difficulty before any "fixing" can start to happen. It's surprising how many areas of information need to be covered to help you develop this understanding of yourself. By the time you've read the last word of this book, you'll have thought about:

- sexual arousal (because most orgasm difficulties are really difficulties in getting highly aroused)
- how to describe and understand an orgasm
- different types of orgasm difficulties (and which type *you* fit into)
- the causes of these different types of orgasm difficulties (and which fit *you*)
- how to change your situation so that you can feel orgasms

Are you wondering if you're ready to take such a close look at yourself? That's understandable. But why not stay with me for a chapter or two (or three) and see how you feel? You may be surprised at some of the tidbits of information that pop out of the coming pages. And, don't forget that having read a few chapters, you can always put the book down and come back to it later when you feel ready.

## types of orgasm difficulties

LET'S BEGIN BY finding out which type of orgasm difficulty you experience. Since the causes of each can be quite different, it's important to know which one you fit into. Let me list these different types for you. Then you can figure out which category seems to fit.

## TYPE ONE: ordinary "garden-variety" orgasm difficulty

Did you know that most women have difficulty reaching orgasm at some time? It really doesn't take much to stop any of us from getting sexually aroused. Stress, tiredness, worry about a child or a parent, or simply not feeling in the mood are examples of some things that can stop us from reaching a sexual climax. So if you occasionally have problems in this area, you're in good company, because there are thousands of women just like you (and me) to whom exactly the same thing happens.

## TYPE TWO: women who never have an orgasm

Perhaps you've never had an orgasm; there are plenty of women who haven't. You may have tried and tried, with no luck. Or, you may have been unaware that women could have such a feeling. Or, you may have never wanted such an experience before now.

## TYPE THREE: women who rarely have an orgasm

Perhaps you occasionally orgasm, but only after what seems like a great deal of hard work on your part—and a lot of luck! For some women it takes a glass of wine and a time of being unusually relaxed for this to happen.

## TYPE FOUR: women who used to be able to orgasm

You may be one of those women who feels quite frustrated because she used to be able to feel orgasms, but can't at the moment. Or, you may be finding that your orgasms have become so weak or so quick that you hardly notice them. Perhaps the ease with which you used to have orgasms has gone and you now struggle to make them happen.

## TYPE FIVE: women who can orgasm at some times, but not others

Then again, you may be able to climax quite easily *except* when you're:

- engaged in a particular kind of sexual practice (such as intercourse), or

- having sex with a partner rather than on your own (don't you wonder how orgasm can be so hard to reach with someone else around, but so easy during masturbation?), or
- having sex with a particular type of person (e.g., a thin man; a gentle woman; someone who's been drinking), or
- having sex with a particular partner (your current partner; someone you've just met).

Did you realize so many types of orgasm difficulties existed? Or that thousands of women fit each of these descriptions? It's true. So, just in case you've been thinking you were an oddity or abnormal, think again. Many, *many* women have exactly the same difficulties you have.

And most of us, as I mentioned earlier, have experienced the Type One variety and found orgasm difficult to feel on occasions (but don't expect it to be a topic of conversation at your next social get-together—we're a bit shy of talking about these things).

---

Okay, so I'm not an oddball. But I am one
VERY frustrated woman when I have sex.
My feelings seem to go so far and stop. . . .
It's like they hit a brick wall.

---

Yep, that's frustrating all right. However, just make sure being frustrated doesn't lead to thinking you're a second-rate woman. Let me explain what I mean.

## feeling negative |

UNFORTUNATELY, SOME WOMEN with orgasm difficulties start to convert their feelings of frustration into negative thoughts about themselves.

- They feel there's something wrong with them, that they're different from other women.
- They believe they aren't good enough because they can't orgasm.

- They see themselves as not being complete women, that something is missing.
- They worry their partner will leave if they don't have an orgasm *soon*.

If you're thinking like this, my guess is you're also feeling (check whichever applies):

❑ miserable
❑ depressed
❑ insecure
❑ unworthy
❑ useless
❑ ashamed
❑ fed up
❑ angry with yourself
❑ something similar to the above _____

The kinds of emotions I've listed here often pop up whenever we start blaming *ourselves* for our orgasm difficulty. This is a great pity. In later chapters, when I begin to identify the causes of orgasm problems, you'll see that there are some very real and logical reasons why women can't orgasm easily. And none of these reasons relate to being a second-rate person.

**What you DO is quite separate from who you ARE.**

Please remember this. Just because you want an orgasm and can't have one (what you *do*) doesn't mean to say you aren't a nice and interesting person (who you *are*). In other words, you can have difficulties with having orgasms and *still* be the kind of person I'd like to get to know.

---

But it's hard to think positive when I've tried
and tried and tried to get highly aroused,
with no success.

---

Maybe it is. Still, think about the determination and strength you've shown to keep going as much as you have. I hope you've got a little of that stamina left to read this book and find out why your past efforts have not brought you the sexual feelings you want.

Stay with me. We're going to explore the causes of arousal difficulties and help you identify which ones seem to fit your situation. I've described *twenty-five* reasons why women have difficulties with orgasm. I'd be surprised if at least one of these didn't explain what happens to you when you begin to get aroused. Then, we'll take a look at what changes can be made so you *can* get aroused enough to orgasm when you want.

If you're having sex (either on your own or with a partner) and thoroughly enjoying it, congratulations! This really makes the point that orgasms are only *one* way of feeling sexual pleasure. And congratulations, too, if you've continued with sex despite being very frustrated and negative at the lack of orgasm. There are women who give up expressing their sexuality because an orgasm seems impossible to achieve. Quite understandable, but a great shame. Hopefully this book will give them the confidence to start feeling sexual again.

## pressure to have orgasms

---

Well, I'm not usually a quitter, but the harder I try to orgasm, the worse things seem to get. It just seems easier not to go through all that hassle.

---

Ah, you've discovered how an orgasm works—or I should say, *doesn't* work. If there is a rule about orgasms, it's this:

**The harder you try to have one, the further away it seems to go.**

In other words, if you keep pushing yourself to make one happen, you'll end up feeling less sexual than when you started (and a whole lot more bad tempered).

It's easy to become so focused on *wanting* an orgasm that it becomes the only reason for being sexual. Orgasm then becomes the *goal* of lovemaking or masturbation (expressing sexual pleasure on your own). But what happens when you can't meet your goal? You feel terrible, a failure, disappointed and so on. You may also feel that you should have an orgasm so as not to disappoint your partner.

Eventually, this pressure becomes too much to bear. Some women cope by pretending to have an orgasm, believing this will please their partner and take the pressure off themselves. Others feel that the only alternative is to switch off from sexual feelings altogether. I suspect neither of these alternatives leaves any woman feeling truly happy.

So let me suggest a truce. *You* take the pressure off yourself. *I'll* try to show you why you can't orgasm at present, and how you can become aroused enough to do so.

**In the meantime, just relax and enjoy the feelings of sexual pleasure you do have.**

Assuming you're now ready to take the pressure off yourself, let's check if there is anyone else pressuring you. It could be a:

❑ husband
❑ partner
❑ girlfriend
❑ lover
❑ fiancé
❑ casual partner
❑ other _____

Take a moment to think about it. Sometimes the reactions of sexual partners can be obvious, such as when annoyance or impatience is expressed because you don't orgasm. Sometimes reactions are more subtle. The following is a true example of one woman's situation. Her partner thought he was being encouraging when he said:

> *Don't worry, honey, I know you'll get there. We'll just keep trying. I'm sure there's something that will help you.*

Did this help? I'm afraid not. All it did was reinforce to "honey" that she needed to find the "right" method (whatever that was). She tried a few things, but began to feel like a circus performer jumping through hoops just so her partner would feel she was trying to "solve the problem." After doing this for a while, she started to avoid sex and to resent her partner.

Some women find the pressure from another person makes them desperate to try *anything* that will help them to "be a normal woman."

---

> Hey, I'd be happy to try anything if I only knew which hoops to jump through. I'd love to find a simple instruction manual, but so far I've had no luck.

---

Well, you're not alone there. Many women with orgasm difficulties don't know what to do (or where to go) to improve things. Some believe that going to a sexual therapist or psychologist would be too embarrassing (or expensive). I've seen women who thought about getting help for years before taking the plunge into counseling. (And some of them cursed loudly when their difficulties disappeared sooner than expected.)

However, some women feel so resentful towards a partner who has been pressuring them that they don't want to make the effort, even if it means helping themselves to feel greater sexual pleasure. And resentment also plays a part for women who believe their partner *should* give them an orgasm and feel annoyed if this doesn't happen.

Have you noticed how resentment makes it awfully hard to be warm and intimate? How can you begin to relax and enjoy yourself during sex if all you feel inside is pent-up anger? With great difficulty!

Resentment is *absolutely* the biggest dampener of sexual arousal in women. And without *strong* sexual feelings, there is no way—*I repeat*, no way—you're ever going to have an orgasm.

So far I've talked about the pressure you get from yourself and from your partner. But let's not forget what little gems society has to offer, too. If you have access to magazines on women's health and sexuality, you'll have probably read headlines something like this:

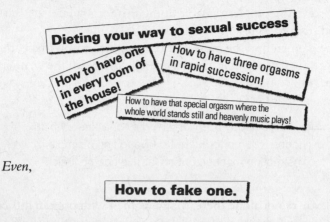

**Dieting your way to sexual success**

**How to have one in every room of the house!**

**How to have three orgasms in rapid succession!**

How to have that special orgasm where the whole world stands still and heavenly music plays!

*Even,*

**How to fake one.**

What a lot of pressure there is to have an orgasm! You'd be forgiven for believing that every woman you meet is able to have one—except you.

Now, remember what I said: there are hundreds and hundreds of women having difficulties just like yours. Your friends may not chat openly about these things, but that doesn't mean they aren't experiencing the same difficulties. Wouldn't it be wonderful if we did talk about these things more honestly? Can you imagine the conversation over coffee?

> *Oh, girls, what a problem I had last night! I sweated my way through sex for two hours and then that damn orgasm just disappeared into thin air. What am I going to do?*

## orgasms aren't everything in sex |

THIS HEADING SHOULD probably be in VERY LARGE print to emphasize how important it is.

----

What, are you crazy?
You write a whole book on how women can have
orgasms, and now you say they aren't important?

----

No, I'm not crazy (well, not in regard to this point, anyway). And I'm not saying that orgasms aren't important to us. But most societies have made such a big deal of having them that it's easy to forget about the enjoyable parts of sex or lovemaking that don't involve orgasm. Such as:

- being physically close with a partner
- having fun
- being relaxed
- feeling the pleasure of sexual arousal inside our body
- allowing ourselves to be held and comforted
- feeling intimate
- being raunchy and letting go
- switching off from work
- feeling sensuous
- feeling cared for

And so on . . .

And if you don't have a partner and like to touch yourself or masturbate, it's equally enjoyable to arouse and caress yourself, to feel your body get turned on, be able to switch off the rest of the world, and to fantasize being touched.

So let's put things back into perspective. Yes, orgasms can be very enjoyable, and it's true women often feel happy being able to express themselves in this way. And, yes, it's great to have the *option* to orgasm, to feel we've been able to express our peak sexual feelings. However, sex can be great without an orgasm.

Having orgasms is *one* of the ways we human beings can feel pleasure and express ourselves sexually. But orgasm shouldn't be the main (or only) focus of our lovemaking. I believe our only goal should be to enjoy the pleasure we can get from expressing ourselves sexually. This pleasure may come through touching, holding, feeling loved, a sexual position, kissing, having fun, and so on. Orgasms may or may not be part of this.

## men can be different

IF YOU HAVE a male partner, you may find he doesn't fully understand my last point. While men can enjoy the intimacy of sex too, they're often less focused on it than women. They're more likely to see an orgasm (and vaginal intercourse) as the goal of sex. Sexual expression is often more important than romance and sensuality (the nice feelings we get when our senses—touch, smell, sound, sight, and taste—are aroused). Many women tend to operate in reverse: they find lovemaking without sensuality and romance to be less emotionally satisfying and less sexually exciting.

If men get turned on or sexually aroused, they're often keen for sexual activity and orgasm to follow soon after. Women, on the other hand, don't always assume, as men often do, that sexual activity and orgasms should follow. They may want to spend a lot of time touching and being close. And, if aroused, they may choose to let their sexual feelings drift away rather than have them become stronger.

The truth is that men often don't understand the whole business of women's difficulties with orgasms. The vast majority of them have experienced orgasm by late teens. Even if they have problems expressing themselves sexually with a partner, most men can easily orgasm during masturbation. No wonder they have trouble empathizing with a woman's difficulties in this area.

## sometimes women are too similar

IF YOUR PARTNER is a woman, you may have a different set of issues to deal with. She may seem really understanding of your difficulties and at no time pressure you about having an orgasm. But something else can happen here. She may be so keen to avoid stressing you that she'll go too far the other way and won't encourage *any* sexual activity at all. This can easily happen. In relationships between women, female needs set the scene. The emphasis on sensuality, cuddling and kissing (common to most women, whoever their partner is) can override the desire for sex or for sexual arousal.

Although this situation may take the pressure off you to orgasm, it can also change the relationship to the extent that you feel like companions rather than lovers.

## how to use this book |

I WANT TO be blunt here and say that not all readers will be able to benefit from *The Elusive Orgasm*. The question of who will and who won't benefit is tackled in chapter 2. I urge you to read this short chapter carefully in order to find out which group you fit into.

Since some women aren't exactly sure what an orgasm *is*, I've used chapter 3 to try to help them. Those of you who have never experienced orgasm or aren't sure whether you have, should find this useful. If you *are* familiar with orgasms, take a few moments to read through the chapter, anyway. Some of the ideas mentioned in it pop up at different times later in the book (for example, the bit about the Arousal Hill). And if you haven't read anything on women's genitals for a while, you may be surprised at what we now know about the clitoris. I imagine there are quite a few of my readers who'll be saying, *"Well, I never knew THAT."* by the end of this chapter.

In chapters 4, 5, and 6, I'll discuss the possible causes of each of the orgasm difficulties, twenty-five in total.

---

Hey, did you say *three* chapters on what causes
orgasm difficulties? And twenty-five causes?
This is beginning to sound serious.

---

Maybe, but each type of orgasm difficulty needs to be given attention. Each of the three chapters will cover different groups of women.

Chapter 4:   Covers women who have never, or only occa-
             sionally, had an orgasm (Types 2 and 3)
Chapter 5:   Covers women who used to be able to have an
             orgasm, but now find it impossible or more dif-
             ficult to do so, or find their orgasm is hardly
             noticeable (Type 4)
Chapter 6:   Covers women who have difficulties only in some
             situations, or with some people and not others
             (Type 5)

Even if you're busy (and who among us is *not?*), I *strongly* recommend that you read through the chapters on each of the different
groups. Sometimes there can be an overlap between the different types.
And you never know which piece of information will suddenly make
you say, "*Uh huh, that seems to fit me, too!*"

By the way, you may find there are several causes of your orgasm difficulties—so don't stop reading just because the first one seems to fit.

From chapter 7 onward, I've outlined ways in which you can overcome the causes of your orgasm difficulties. Now . . .

HOLD IT!

I know it's tempting to dash ahead, but remember, if you want to
choose the right treatment approach, you must first find out what it
is that stops you from having orgasms. There's absolutely no point trying to change things if you don't know exactly what it is you have
to change.

**Oh, and one more thing:** throughout the book I'll be asking
questions, giving you a quiz or two and offering exercises you
might like to try. I suggest you write down your answers as well as
any thoughts you want to record. You may like to use a notebook
or the pages at the end of this book. A notebook is also essential if
you've borrowed this book from a library and need to leave it clean
for the next reader.

# but first,
# are you ready
# to orgasm?

T HERE are two important questions which need to be answered before you tackle the rest of the book. This chapter will help you to work out your response to each one. Here are the questions:

**Question 1:** Do you actually have a problem with orgasm?

**Question 2:** Are you ready to look at why you have orgasm difficulties?

If you find that the answer to either question is no, it's unlikely that your orgasm difficulties will be helped by *The Elusive Orgasm*. So, let's check whether I'm going to be able to help you. Better to do this now than to be disappointed later.

# CHECK #1:
## which problem is it?

> Listen, I KNOW when I can't orgasm. How could
> anyone be confused about what the problem is?

Well, of course, most woman know quite clearly when they can or can't orgasm. But for some women, the *real* problem is that *they don't feel any sexual desire.* Let me try and explain this further.

To have an orgasm we have to be feeling highly aroused sexually. I mean, *really* aroused or "turned on." These feelings of sexual pleasure seem to center on our genital area, but can also be felt in other parts of our body. Now here's the interesting bit: women with orgasm problems usually have *no* difficulty feeling sexual desire or getting aroused to some level. . . .

**They just don't get aroused ENOUGH to experience orgasm.**

Women who feel very little or no sexual desire have a different problem. They simply don't have an interest in sex. If you feel no interest in expressing yourself sexually, you won't be in the mood to get aroused or be willing to try. If you don't get aroused, you won't orgasm.

If this describes you, it's likely that you never think about being sexual (on your own or with a partner), and can happily leave the whole sex business to others without feeling you're missing out on a thing. Or, you may find yourself in the mood on rare occasions, helped along by a glass of wine or an exciting new partner. *And when this happens you may find you can orgasm quite easily.*

Therefore, you don't really have a difficulty with orgasm. Rather, your real difficulty is with not feeling enough sexual interest or desire to encourage you into situations where you become aroused and experience an orgasm.

It's important to understand that **lack of sexual desire** is a related but *different* kind of sexual problem from **difficulty with orgasm**. While this book has not been written specifically for women who lack an interest in sex, I believe it may still be useful in helping you to understand a little more about yourself. The causes of lack of sexual interest are often different from those of orgasm difficulties, but there is some similarity. So, the information provided in the next few chapters may be useful and offer something for you to think about.

The same thing applies to the Change Programs outlined in later chapters for women with orgasm difficulties. Some sections may be helpful, while others will not be suitable for women who lack sexual desire.

I must point out, however, that both kinds of problems can be connected. For example, women who start out with good levels of sexual desire can become so frustrated with their difficulty in experiencing orgasm that they eventually lose all interest in sex. And, as I mentioned earlier, women who usually have no sexual desire may easily have orgasms on the occasions when they do engage in sexual activity.

# CHECK #2: |
## can you be bothered?

DO YOU REALLY care about having an orgasm or not? I'm sure one or two of you are reading this book only because a lover/ex-partner/friend gave it to you as a gift (a rather unsubtle hint?). Perhaps you're reading through it quickly just so you can say,

> *Yes, nice little book. Quite useful, I suppose. I might try some of the suggestions when I have more time. . . .*

Maybe you were hoping I'd offer some quick-fix solution in the first chapter, so that your partner is kept happy without you having to do too much yourself. That probably means you're not really interested in having orgasms for yourself.

Then again, perhaps you're motivated to read what I have to say *only* because you think it will improve your relationship. You may believe it will keep the peace, bring you closer or help to sort out other problems you have. Maybe you feel guilty about not being able to please your partner who, you know, would like you to be able to orgasm.

There are many women who simply can't see what all the fuss is about. And the truth is, there *is* far too much fuss made of the whole topic of having an orgasm.

**But what about your needs? Do you care one way or the other about your own pleasure?**

Of course, if you've never had an orgasm and can't begin to imagine what it's like to have one, then you're hardly likely to get excited, are you? Picture what would happen if you rushed up to a group of people who'd never heard of or tasted ice cream and told them they should try it. Are they going to jump up with glee and race off to the nearest store? Hardly!

Well, orgasms aren't much different. It's perfectly understandable if you're not sure what all the fuss is about. Even those of you who used to experience orgasms may have forgotten how nice it was to orgasm easily and without pressure.

So, the question is, how keen are you to understand why you can't orgasm? And, how enthusiastic are you about learning (or relearning) how to orgasm? Are you really interested or just half-hearted?

---

Well look, how long can a person
keep on trying before they lose interest?

---

Good question! It *is* hard to stay keen. Yet, without the desire to *try*—and I mean try for *you*—I'm afraid you probably won't get very far along the Programs offered later in this book.

If you're feeling half-hearted about the whole situation, be honest with yourself about your lack of motivation and wait until you're willing to try again. And remember,

**You don't have to orgasm—or even want to.**

You don't even have to read another chapter in this book: so, don't feel pressured to do so. *But* . . . (I'm sure you knew there would be a "but . . ."):

All I ask is that, before tucking this book away in the bookcase, you consider *why* you don't want to orgasm. I'm not saying you *should* orgasm. I simply want you to think about and understand your reaction.

Is your decision based on something positive, such as wanting to put all your energy into a special project at the moment? That may be fine, unless this is something you always do. Do you always throw yourself into completing tasks at the expense of taking time for yourself? Is there a lack of balance between work and play, or between "doing for me" and "doing for others"? Do you give time to your relationship only when all the tasks are finished?

Then ask yourself whether having an orgasm is important enough. If it's down the bottom of your list of "things to do," you'll probably never feel ready to follow the suggestions made in later chapters. There'll always be something else more important to do.

Perhaps your half-heartedness is related to something you want to avoid, such as fear of failure, anger with your partner, nervousness at being vulnerable. Again, be honest with yourself about this. After all, it's perfectly acceptable to want to avoid a situation which threatens to make you feel terrible.

Now consider whether you would like to try and feel orgasms if only you could get over your fear, embarrassment, resentment, nervousness, and so on. If your answer is yes, maybe a chat with a friendly psychologist will help you through these emotions and free you up to do what you secretly want to do.

Sometimes it can be poor health, rather than emotions, that stops women from feeling motivated to try and have orgasms. If you have been or are currently ill, you may not feel well enough to do anything about your orgasm difficulty. In that case, be kind to yourself and stop worrying about having orgasms. Wait until you have more energy and interest. Let me tell you, trying to work through the Change Programs will be no fun if you're feeling unwell. There are no medals for orgasmic martyrdom, I'm afraid!

☙

SO THEN, CHECK out why you may be half-hearted about trying to have an orgasm. Don't let yourself become pressured into following the Programs outlined in my book unless you feel ready to do so.

But, keep in mind that it *is* nice to have the *option* to choose whether to have an orgasm or not. Knowing *how to* orgasm doesn't mean you *have to* orgasm.

And finally, let me remind you of something I said in chapter 1. There are many women who are quite content with not having orgasms. I've worked with plenty for whom sex was great fun—without their feeling a single orgasm.

# 3

# what is orgasm?

TRYING to describe an orgasm is like trying to describe the joy of sinking into bed after a busy day, or the exquisiteness of a particularly beautiful sunset, or the delight of swimming in the sea on a hot afternoon. It's impossible to put feelings like these into words.

Women who haven't experienced an orgasm often feel embarrassed by their inability to say what it is.

---

Well, everyone seems to know about orgasms
except me. I'm too ashamed to say anything, but I
don't have a clue what an orgasm is. It's like I'm
supposed to know!

---

It's true. We're all supposed to know what an orgasm is. But who gives us this information? Our parents? Heavens, no! Our school friends? Unlikely. Our teachers or sex educators? Rarely. They seem to skip over anything to do with sexual arousal. And, most of us aren't comfortable, as adults, asking a friend or partner.

Interestingly, when I checked the word *orgasm* in my computer's dictionary, I was told, NO SUGGESTIONS AVAILABLE. That's odd, because my computer immediately informs me when I spell the word incorrectly.

Various dictionaries declare,

**"Orgasm is the climax of sexual excitement."**

Does that make you any the wiser? I doubt it.

Some would say you can't know what orgasms are until you experience at least one. I guess it's like chocolate: only when you taste it can you really understand what it is. The truth is most people *do* learn about orgasms by having one.

---

But if I'm not able to climax, and everyone just
assumes I know what orgasms are, AND the whole
business of explaining them is so difficult, how am I
ever going to move on? I seem to be stuck.

---

You're not alone in feeling this way, believe me. For women who have never experienced orgasm, the whole thing can seem a real mystery. While I can't give you the actual experience, in this chapter I'd like to help you unravel the mystery a little.

Even if you have felt an orgasm, there's probably a great deal about arousal and orgasm that's still a mystery. So, read on and find out what your parents, teachers and friends weren't able to tell you.

## what is sexual arousal? |

AS I MENTIONED in chapter 1, to understand orgasms we need to understand sexual arousal.

**Difficulties with orgasm, you may recall, are really difficulties in getting highly aroused.**

Let me talk, then, about *sexual arousal*. Unfortunately, sexual arousal (or getting "turned on") is no easier to define than orgasm. The simplest explanation is to describe it as feelings of pleasure that seem to center in our genitals and spread throughout other parts of our body.

We often experience these pleasurable sensations as different from other feelings of enjoyment, but it's hard to put this difference into words. Sexual pleasure seems to feel *more* exquisite, *more* intense, and *more* focused on areas of our body that we know as sexual areas. These feelings of pleasure are caused by temporary changes in our body, thoughts, and emotions. In this chapter, I want to help you understand these amazing changes as a first step towards understanding your orgasm difficulties.

## sexual triggers—learning what is arousing |

SEXUAL AROUSAL BEGINS when some event, object, or person sexually excites us or stimulates our interest in sex. Learning what is sexually exciting is part of what we learn while growing up. Strange as it may seem, we aren't born with an understanding of what is "sexual" or what is "sexually exciting." It comes from our culture, upbringing, and life experiences.

Let's not forget, however, that baby girls can show physical signs of arousal. Now they certainly haven't learned whether something is sexual or not, so what's going on? Well, touching their genitals appears to trigger a feeling of pure pleasure. Someone else might think of it as "sexual pleasure," but to the little girls it's just a good feeling they get. It has no sexual meaning.

When we're older, touch is also an important trigger to feelings of pleasure. But it's what that touch *means* to us (what we think and feel about it) that is just as important as the actual contact—maybe even *more* important.

However, touch is only one of the many things that can start you feeling sexually aroused. Without even realizing it, you've been developing a whole set of *sexual triggers*, things that get you thinking about, and feeling, sexual. Sexual triggers focus your attention on sexual topics and begin to arouse you. They're learned as we're growing up and right through adulthood.

It's important to understand your sexual triggers, because they're the first step to getting aroused (and eventually having an orgasm). Take a few moments to try the quiz on this and the next page. It should help you to identify your sexual triggers.

## your sexual triggers

1. What kinds of **touch** are sexually exciting to you?
   *(For example, a flirtatious, teasing touch)*

   _____

   _____

2. What kinds of **smells** are sexually exciting to you?
   *(For example, perfume or body odor)*

   _____

   _____

3. What kinds of **sounds** are sexually exciting to you?
   *(For example, someone moaning with pleasure)*

   _____

   _____

4. What kinds of **sights** are sexually exciting to you?
   *(For example, catching a glimpse of a person you find "attractive")*

   _____

   _____

5. What kinds of **tastes** are sexually exciting to you?
   *(For example, the taste of salty skin)*

   _____

   _____

6. What **types of people** are sexually exciting to you?
   *(For example, black-haired people with a sense of humor)*

   _____

   _____

7. What **types of objects** are sexually exciting to you?
   *(For example, silky underwear)*

   _____

   _____

8. What **types of situations** are sexually exciting to you?
   *(For example, a romantic dinner)*

   _____

   _____

9. What kinds of **thoughts** are sexually exciting to you?
   *(For example, thinking you might have sex later that day)*

   _____

   _____

I should mention that sometimes our reactions to sexual triggers are so fast that we aren't immediately conscious of what's happening. It's only when we notice our body reacting that we realize something or someone has stimulated us to feel sexually aroused.

No two people are alike in what arouses them. Your set of sexual triggers will be different from those of other women. You might, for example, find a catchy grin really sexy, but another woman may not even notice it.

> That's all very well, but having my breasts touched doesn't trigger anything. Since I know other woman get turned on by this, there must be something wrong with me.

No, there's nothing wrong with you. There are many women whose sexual feelings aren't triggered when their breasts are stroked. This may simply be the way you are. Perhaps other parts of your body (for example, your back) are better triggers for your arousal if touched in a way you think is "romantic" or "sexy." Or, there may be a good reason why you don't feel sexually excited when your breasts are touched. For example, an unknown man may have grabbed your breast in an unpleasant way when you were younger. This kind of experience leaves some women with a general dislike of being touched on the breast.

**And another thing:** women often find that sexual triggers vary from day to day. Something that triggers arousal one day may be less exciting on another day. It all depends on our mood, what's happening in our lives, where we are in our menstrual cycle, and so on.

Interestingly, many women find their arousal is more easily triggered at certain times of their menstrual cycle (often just before, during, or after a period). You might check whether this happens for you.

As you can see, becoming sexually excited depends on our physical and psychological (mental and emotional) reactions, as well as on what's happening in the world around us. No one could accuse us of being staid and predictable, could they?

# building sexual arousal

THE LONGER WE'RE able to stay in the situation that triggers our feelings of sexual pleasure, the more intense those feelings will become. Building the level of sexual pleasure is important because, well . . . for one thing, the feelings are *sooo* nice.

**It's also the path to feeling orgasms.**

A woman's feelings of sexual pleasure will usually get stronger if:

- She is aware of what she needs to build the feelings and is able to ask for this from a partner or to do this for herself.
- The sexually sensitive areas of her body are touched (by herself or a partner) in the way that suits her at the time.
- She feels positive about herself.
- She feels positive about her partner.
- She feels safe in the sexual situation.
- She feels positive about the sexual situation.
- She accepts the image of herself as a sexual being.
- She has no injury or physical condition preventing her from building arousal.

With all these conditions needing to be met, it's not surprising that some women find it more difficult to build their sexual arousal than do others.

# understanding the physical side of arousal |

I'LL BE TALKING about each of these conditions throughout the next few chapters. Right now, let me spend some time on the second condition: the touching of those parts of a woman's body which help to build her arousal.

---

Oh, do you mean genitals and all that stuff? Then I could probably skip the section. I read a couple of books when I was younger. I mean, how many pictures of vaginas can you look at?

---

I understand what you're saying. However, did you know that our understanding of women's genitals, *especially the clitoris*, has changed quite a bit in the last ten years or so? Perhaps you should check whether your ideas are up to date. I promise you quite a bit more than "pictures of vaginas."

Let me begin with the word *genitals*.

## GENITALS

Many women use this term to mean "down there" or "between my legs," but aren't too clear about what it is exactly. I'll use *genitals* to include the areas *inside* and *outside* our body that relate to sexual reactions. The parts outside our body include: the vulva, parts of the clitoris, the vaginal entrance, the urethral opening, the perineum, and the anus. The organs inside our body include: parts of the clitoris, bulbs of the clitoris, the vagina, the urethra and urethral sponge, the perineal sponge, and the uterus.

Now let's check the meaning of the words *vulva*, *clitoris* and *vagina*. It's amazing how confused people get about these terms.

## VULVA

*Vulva* means "covering" or "wrapping." In the past, it was used to describe all the areas of a woman's genitals that are outside her body. But there were problems with this description. Firstly, it is really only the pubic mound and outer lips (labia majora) which act as a "covering."

Secondly, the clitoris is much more important to women's sexuality than other "outside" areas, and this fact tends to get lost when we refer to everything as "the vulva." While it was easy to use a single word (*vulva*) to mean all the outside "bits," this was also another way of making the clitoris less significant than it is. Can you imagine men having one word to cover all their outer "bits" and never talking about their penis? Neither can I! Women need to be just as positive about their clitoris—which, by the way, is physically similar to the penis.

Most importantly, the clitoris has parts on the outside and inside of the body. So it doesn't make sense to use the word *vulva* (which applies only to the outside of the body) to include the clitoris.

I'll be using *vulva* in the modern sense, to mean the **outer lips (or labia majora)** and the **pubic mound** (see figure 1). The outer lips are covered in hair and are sensitive to touch. I'm sure you know this already. Did you also know they contain many small blood vessels which fill with blood when a women is sexually aroused? This makes the lips expand and grow darker in color.

## CLITORIS

This word has an old and a new meaning, too. In the past, *clitoris* was applied to the small round "magic button" or glans of the clitoris—as if that were the whole organ. Even today, many people still believe this. Thanks to some dedicated women researchers, however, we now know this is *wrong, wrong,* WRONG.

There are actually many parts to the clitoris, some of which are *outside* and some of which are *inside* the body. Let's see how many you know about.

I'll briefly describe each of these parts, beginning with *those you can see*. Use figure 1 to find out where each is located.

The clitoris starts where the inner lips connect with the outer lips and pubic mound. The **inner lips** are called the **labia minora**, which means "minor lips," because they are smaller than the outer lips. However, they're *more* important to our sexual arousal than the outer lips. The inner lips are hairless and sensitive to touch. When you're aroused, they swell with blood and become even more sensitive.

Being the interesting creatures that women are, our inner lips (and outer lips as well) vary greatly in shape and colors. In fact, no two women are ever the same. Oh, and don't worry if one side of your labia differs in size or shape from the other. This is also *very* common (but distressing for the perfectionists among us). Some women think they look odd because of these differences. If that's the case, we must *all* look odd! I prefer to think that the way each woman looks is just *right* for her.

The inner lips join near the pubic mound to form a tent-shaped **hood** over the **glans, or head, of the clitoris** (a bit like the hood of a raincoat). The **hood of the clitoris** protects the glans in the same way as the foreskin protects the glans of a man's penis. The hood also protects the **shaft of the clitoris**.

The **glans of the clitoris** is *extremely* sensitive. And no wonder, with somewhere between 6,000 and 8,000 nerve endings crowding one small area. Not surprisingly, the purpose of the clitoris glans *is simply to create feelings of pleasure*.

The glans is made of an erectile tissue (*corpus spongiosum*) that consists of many, many tiny spaces (as in a sponge), arteries, and veins. The spaces fill with blood (as a sponge gets filled with water) when a woman is sexually aroused. This makes the glans swell and become firmer.

For many women, the clitoris glans is so sensitive that it feels more like an *ouch* rather than an *oooh* if touched directly. No wonder it needs a hood for protection. And one more thing: one side of the clitoris glans often feels more sensitive than the other (a source of frustration to partners who haven't learned which side is which!).

Between the clitoral glans and the **entrance of the vagina** lies the **opening of the urethra**, the tube from which we urinate.

Now, let me turn to the parts of the clitoris *inside* the body (figure 2).

I'll begin with the **shaft, or body, of the clitoris**. This joins the glans and is also very sensitive. It's usually about three-quarters to one-and-a-half inches (two to four centimeters) long and three-eights to three-quarters inches (one to two centimeters) wide, and is made up of a different kind of erectile tissue (*corpus cavernosum*) from the glans.[4] The cavernosum tissue also has many spaces (like little caves), as well as tiny arteries and veins. These spaces fill with blood when a woman is aroused, making the shaft swell. It then becomes quite firm and raised, or *erect* (See figure 3).

This is why we call it *erectile* tissue. Both spongiosum and cavernosum tissue cause swelling, firmness, and erection, but cavernosum tissue gives a firmer erection.

---

Wait a minute. Just wait a minute! Do you mean to tell me that WOMEN have erections? Just like men?

---

Yes, that's exactly what I'm saying. The clitoris is the sexual organ that swells and gets erect during sexual arousal, although it doesn't get quite as hard as a man's penis. Haven't noticed your erection? Don't worry. A woman's erection happens inside her body and can't be clearly seen, as it can on a man. However, some parts of the erection can be felt through the skin—as you'll soon learn.

It's not just the shaft and glans of the clitoris that swell, either. There are other areas that also become erect when you're turned on. Keep reading to find out what these are.

The clitoris continues from the shaft, dividing into two branches or **legs of the clitoris**, also known as **crura**. The legs are an amazing two- to three-and-a-half inches (five to nine centimeters) long and lie under the inner lips, along the pelvic bones.[5] They fan out from the shaft like a wishbone, one on either side of the urethral and vaginal openings. To see how this looks from a front view, turn to figure 4.

The legs of the clitoris, or crura, are made of the same erectile tissue as the shaft, so they'll also fill with blood and become hard and erect when a woman gets turned on.

ॐ

NOW, LET ME stop for a minute so you can catch your breath. Many women have been taught that the clitoris is just a little "button" or "pea," tiny in size. *And, here I am telling you that the clitoris is actually much longer*—about two and three-quarters to five and one-eighth inches (seven to thirteen centimeters)—when we include the glans, shaft, and legs.

Isn't that great news? There's just so much more of the clitoris to get sexual pleasure from.

℘

BUT, WAIT FOR it . . . there's *more*. I haven't finished describing the clitoris.

Lying underneath the inner lips and looking a bit like two triangle-shaped pendants are the **bulbs of the clitoris** (figures 2 to 4). They surround the upper side of the urethra before branching off into two . . . well, bulbs. If you're standing, they slope down slightly towards the ground, while the clitoral legs point backwards towards your buttocks.

The bulbs are made up of the same kind of spongy erectile tissue (*corpus spongiosum*) as the glans. When you're sexually turned on, the bulbs swell, becoming firmer and erect. It's thought this might help to stiffen the walls of the vagina, making penetration easier.

*Another* area of this spongy erectile tissue surrounds the urethra and is sometimes called the **urethral sponge** or female prostate. Within this tissue are many tiny glands (about thirty or more), two of which (Skene's Glands) are found near the urethral opening. These thirty or more glands, called the **paraurethral** and **periurethral glands**, produce a fluid similar to male prostatic fluid.

This fluid is thought to be the source of *women's ejaculation* (release of fluid), something I know is of interest to many women. I'll talk more about ejaculation shortly.

When a woman is sexually turned on, the urethral sponge fills with blood, making it swell and become erect. A section of this erect tissue can then be felt through the vaginal wall. We call this the **Grafenberg spot** or **G-spot**. It's not really a spot, but actually a small area of the vaginal wall resting against the urethral sponge. When a woman is aroused, the swollen sponge pushes against the wall. For many women, this area becomes very sensitive.

If stroked during sexual arousal (by a finger, penis, dildo, vibrator, and so on), the G-spot can increase the strength of our sexual feelings. However, this doesn't happen for all women. Some women find their G-spot isn't very sensitive. This may be because they don't get fully aroused. Or, it may be just the way they are.

The G-spot can be found about a finger-length inside the vagina by pressing up towards your pubic bone. It may be easier to find if you draw your knees up close to your chest. But, don't forget, you need to be sexually excited to make the G-spot noticeable.

Touching of the G-spot (really the urethral sponge) can also lead to ejaculation. However, there are many women who ejaculate with touch to the clitoris glans and shaft, rather than the G-spot.

Ejaculation is a squirt of fluid that comes out of the urethra, usually at the point of orgasm. IT ISN'T URINE. I've put this in capital letters because some women worry that they're "wetting the bed" or urinating. You're not!

**You're simply expressing your sexual excitement.**

The amount ejaculated can be as little as a few drops or as much as a cupful. It's likely that all women ejaculate. So, if you think you don't ejaculate, think again. It may be that the amount is simply too small for you to notice.

Just below the vaginal opening there are two more glands lying beneath the skin. These are called the **vulvovaginal glands** or **Bartholin's glands**. When a woman is aroused, they produce a few drops of thick fluid that help to wet the opening of the vagina.

Underneath the **perineum** (the skin between the vaginal opening and the anus) is another area which becomes erect during sexual arousal. This is called the **perineal sponge**, and it's made up of a tightly packed bundle of blood vessels and erectile tissue. When you're aroused, the perineal sponge fills with blood, swells, and become firmer. This makes the perineum highly sensitive. For some women, any touch or pressure to this area can be felt deep in the stomach area. By the way, the perineum is often cut during childbirth. This may result in damage to the erectile tissue and nerves.

## THE PELVIC MUSCLES

The muscles in our pelvic area play an important role in arousal and orgasm. Because of this, they're seen as part of the whole clitoris system and are sometimes called the clitoral muscles.

There are several layers of muscle, and it may help you to know where these are (see figure 5). Later, I'll talk about what happens to them when you feel sexually aroused.

Let's begin with the *outer layer* of pelvic muscle. It includes the **bulbocavernosus muscle**, the **ischiocavernosus muscle**, and the **transverse perineal muscle**. They lie just underneath the skin in the area between your legs, and the glans, shaft, and legs of the clitoris are surrounded by them. This is a good clue as to why they're important to orgasm—but more on that in the next section.

Underneath the ischiocavernosus and transverse perineal muscles lies the **urogenital diaphragm**, which is the *middle layer* of pelvic muscle. The vagina and the urethra both pass through this flat muscle, which is shaped like a triangle.

The bulbs, legs, and perineal sponge of the clitoris lie between the outer and middle layers of muscle.

The *inner layer* of pelvic muscle lies deeper in the pelvis, underneath all the muscles just described. It's called the **pelvic diaphragm** because it covers the whole pelvic area. The **pubococcygeus** or **PC muscle** (also called *levator ani*) is an important part of this muscle. Women who have a noticeable ejaculation usually have very strong pubococcygeus muscles (so now you can brag about how fit you are).

The pelvic diaphragm runs from the pubic bone to the tail bone and is attached on each side to the pelvic bones. All parts of the clitoris rest on it, and the urethra, urethral sponge, vagina, and anus all go through it.

## PELVIC LIGAMENTS

Another important piece of the clitoris puzzle is the movement of **pelvic ligaments** (the **round ligament** and the **suspensory ligament**). These link the clitoris with other parts of a woman's pelvis, such as the uterus. During arousal and orgasm, movement in the clitoris sends pleasurable "shivers" to these other areas.

## NERVES AND BLOOD VESSELS

**Networks of nerves** and **networks of blood vessels** are two important areas of the clitoris system.

Nerves play an important part in allowing messages from the brain to reach the genitals. These messages give the signal to start the process of arousal. One network of nerves sends sexual messages between the genitals and the brain via the spinal cord. Another network of nerves, running through the intestine, links the uterus to the brain. One of these intestinal nerves, the *vagus nerve*, appears able to send sexual messages to the brain in women whose lower spinal cord is damaged.

Blood vessels are also extremely important to sexual arousal. Arteries bring blood to the hundreds of tiny "spaces" that make up the erectile tissue of the clitoris. This makes the tissue swell and become firm. Veins then carry blood away from the clitoris after orgasm.

## VAGINA

The **vagina** is part of the reproductive system and is a tube linking the outer genitals with the uterus. Although it's not part of the clitoris, it plays a role in sexual arousal in two ways. Firstly, as I mentioned before, it's a way to reach the urethral sponge. And, secondly, at the end of the vagina is the **cervix**, a small opening that leads into the uterus or womb. Some women find that rhythmical pressure on the cervix (by a penis, dildo, or vibrator) is important for them to orgasm. The **uterus** is made up of very strong muscles that contract during orgasm. Its lining also swells with blood during sexual arousal. This helps the feelings of sexual pleasure to spread throughout the whole pelvis.

A final point: some people use the word "vagina" when they are really talking about the "genitals," "vulva" or "clitoris." Hopefully, you now know the meaning of each of these terms and won't be confused any longer.

❦

So THERE YOU have it. Can you now see how the clitoris is much, much more than a little "button"? When you're aroused, the entire clitoris system becomes involved, even if you're not aware of it.

Any one of our sexual triggers can stimulate the clitoris. However, most women need the clitoral glans and shaft to be touched if their arousal is to become stronger and stronger. This shouldn't surprise you. Remember, these areas are extremely sensitive to touch.

In fact, most women find the glans *too* sensitive to touch directly and prefer touching the side of the glans through the hood, or above the glans on the shaft.

The easiest way to feel the shaft is by moving your fingers over the hood in a back-and-forth or round-and-round action. The shaft feels like a short piece of cord and will move from side to side when pressed.

However, while stroking of the glans and shaft are important to building arousal, there are actually many different ways in which women like to be touched.

**There's no right or wrong way to build sexual arousal, only YOUR way.**

Look at some of the different ways that women enjoy physical touch:

- a preference for *only* the outer areas of the clitoris to be touched
- an enjoyment of the outer clitoral areas being touched *and* something pressed inside the vagina
- wanting *only* vaginal penetration
- enjoying the glans and shaft being stroked by fingers (or maybe a feather!)
- enjoying the glans and shaft being stroked by a soft, wet tongue
- enjoying the glans and shaft being stimulated by the pressure of another body or object, such as a vibrator or dildo
- loving anything that vibrates against the clitoris (such as the jet from a spa or shower, or the quick movements of a vibrator)
- wanting the stroking of nipples (because nipples are also made up of sensitive erectile tissue and can be an important part of building arousal)
- needing an area near the cervix (the entrance to the uterus) to be pressed firmly with a penis, vibrator, or dildo (because it can be highly sensitive and very arousing for some women)
- squeezing the pelvic muscles to increase the pleasurable clitoral sensations

- tightening their legs together so the outer clitoris and vulva are squeezed
- enjoying the caressing of skin, because our entire body becomes sensitive when we are aroused.

I should explain the meaning of *vibrator* and *dildo*, for those of you who aren't familiar with these words.

A *vibrator* is an object, made of hard or soft plastic or silicon, that vibrates by electrical current. Vibrators come in many different shapes, sizes and colors. They may use either batteries or electrical power. When pressed against your clitoris or placed inside the vagina, a vibrator can be very arousing because of its strong and steady rhythm.

A *dildo* is a cone-shaped object that varies in length, thickness, color, and texture. It's usually made of a soft material such as silicon or rubber. Dildos do not vibrate, but can create pleasurable sensations if pressed against your clitoris or moved in the vagina or anus.

# becoming aroused |

## PHYSICAL CHANGES

As we build sexual arousal, many physical changes take place. You'll notice some of these changes, but not all of them.

When something or someone acts as a sexual trigger, we start to experience physical changes. Messages are sent by our senses to the brain. The brain reacts by sending several sexual chemicals and hormones into the bloodstream. *As long as we don't try to switch off the sexual triggers*, our bodies begin to react. (This last point is very important, and I'll be talking a lot more about it in later chapters).

Further messages are sent from our brain by nerves to tell the erectile tissue of the clitoris to relax. When this happens, the spaces in the tissue appear. Blood then flows into our clitoris and fills these spaces. The clitoris becomes swollen, firm, and erect. Our lips or labia expand in size and take on a dark pink tinge because of this extra blood in the tissues. Quite pretty, if you take the time to look!

Soon after we become sexually excited, pressure from blood in the cavities of the erectile tissue close to the vaginal walls forces clear fluid through the walls of the vagina. This fluid lubricates or wets the vaginal walls and is called **vaginal lubricant**. The vulvovaginal glands near the entrance to the vagina also create a small amount of fluid for lubrication. These lubricants make it easier to move something (penis, fingers, vibrator, dildo) in the vagina.

However, in women who are menopausal (and not on hormone replacement therapy), the low levels of estrogen in their bodies may stop lubrication occurring, no matter *how* aroused they feel. Of course, they may show many other signs of being physically aroused.

By now, our clitoris glans has become extremely sensitive and erect. To protect it, the suspensory ligament tightens and pulls the glans underneath the hood. Now, that's smart!

The clitoris shaft feels quite hard and round. The clitoris legs have become rigid and longer. The spongy tissue of the bulbs has expanded and pushed out the inner lips and vulva so they also look swollen. The bulbs tighten around the vaginal opening, and this helps to close the entrance of the vagina a little more snugly. The urethral sponge swells and can be felt through the nearby vaginal wall at the G-spot. In some women the sponge may even be seen through the opening of the vagina. The perineal sponge also swells with blood and increases in sensitivity.

We feel our skin become sensitive and tingly as the nerves get stimulated. Our nipples become firm, especially if touched, and send a message to the brain to release more oxytocin, the hormone that gives our vulva and clitoris a nice, tingling feeling.

The first third of the vagina near the opening also swells. The rest of the vagina (deep inside) opens out like a balloon as the round ligament tightens and pulls on the uterus. At the other end, the round ligament pulls on the inner lips, increasing the sensations of sexual pleasure.

The uterus lining becomes swollen with blood and contracts. For those women who feel this happening, it can be a pleasurable sensation.

Not surprisingly, with all this going on, our breathing rate gets faster and so, too, does our heart rate.

As long as you continue to be sexually stimulated by any of your sexual triggers, arousal builds. The muscles also become involved. All the pelvic muscles begin to tighten and this gives a pleasant feeling of tension. As they press against the clitoral tissue, the pleasurable sexual feelings are increased. The tension gets stronger and stronger, and so do the feelings of pleasure.

At the same time, your brain continues to be filled with sexual chemicals that add to the feelings of pleasure.

# becoming aroused |

## PSYCHOLOGICAL CHANGES

Physical changes aren't the only ones taking place. As we begin to get aroused, there are also shifts in our thoughts, emotions, and actions (our psychology).

Our thoughts and emotions turn more and more to sexual matters. We begin to notice the presence of sexual triggers. We begin to get ... IN THE MOOD. Our attention narrows down, shifting from day-to-day events to our sexual feelings. We begin to look forward to experiencing sexual pleasure, although a short time before, we may not have given this a single thought.

Our attitudes, or what we think *about* sexual activities and sexual pleasure, are a very important part of building sexual arousal. Why? Because positive attitudes will help you to focus on the enjoyable moments that are occurring. You'll want to continue the good feelings. Memories (thoughts) of enjoyable sexual moments that happened previously can add to this desire. As you begin to get aroused, good memories help you to feel ready and open to repeating these nice experiences.

Thinking we're attractive to another person also plays a part in building arousal. Believing you're attractive and desired by another person helps you to focus on your feelings of sexual pleasure. This can lead you to feel *more* aroused. The more aroused you are, the more you focus on the aspects of your partner that are attractive to you. Remember, the attractiveness of your partner can be a powerful sexual trigger.

Emotional changes also occur as we become aroused. You feel more vulnerable, happier, affectionate, and so on. You are relaxed and feel closer to your partner. You act more freely and are more playful. You begin to have fun.

❧

PSYCHOLOGICAL AND PHYSICAL changes can happen together. As our body begins to be triggered to physical arousal, we start to think about what's happening. Noticing and thinking about the situation is an important part of the way women get sexually turned on. They like to take a little time to decide whether they're happy to have their feelings triggered in this way, whether they want to be in the present sexual situation, whether they want to take it further, and whether they'll be safe. If everything is okay, they'll feel positive about their feelings of sexual pleasure and begin to feel more turned on.

What we think, feel, and do can *then* cause greater physical changes of arousal. At the same time, physical changes lead to changes in thoughts, emotions, and actions. As physical and psychological changes affect each other, our arousal starts to get stronger.

For most women, however, there are many occasions when the two types of changes *don't happen at the same time.*

---

That seems to fit me. Sometimes when my partner says I'm wet in the vagina, I don't feel a thing. She thinks I'm aroused, but I'm not. Who's right?

---

You both are! Women often show physical signs of being turned on (such as getting wet in the vagina) but don't notice or recognize these signs for what they are—sexual arousal. Because of this they're not ready for sex or in the mood. They don't feel sexy in their thoughts or emotions (there are no psychological changes), so don't see themselves as turned on.

Perhaps they haven't had time to relax and switch off from a busy day. Maybe they see the physical changes as irritating because their minds are filled with worrying thoughts. Perhaps they don't know how to recognize physical changes related to sexual arousal.

On the other hand, women can sometimes think sexy thoughts and feel in the mood, but their bodies don't show any signs of arousal. Let me give you an example of this. After drinking a few glasses of alcohol, women often feel quite turned on. But, the truth is, their physical signs of arousal can decrease as a result of this amount of alcohol.

## from high sexual arousal to orgasm |

IF WE STAY for a time in a situation where the changes in our bodies and minds come together—and we enjoy this—our arousal will build. The feelings of sexual pleasure will grow stronger and stronger and we'll feel ourselves climbing higher and higher towards a peak of sexual arousal.

The orgasm is the *highest point* or *peak* of our sexual arousal. Because of this, it's a particularly pleasurable feeling, what I would call a "burst of pleasure." Some people refer to it as a *climax*, another word for "peak." A popular term in English is also *coming*, a shorthand way of talking about "coming to the peak of arousal."

**Reaching orgasm is similar to climbing a hill.**

You keep climbing and climbing, enjoying the scenery along the way. As you get closer to the top, you increase your pace, wanting to see what's at the top. Suddenly, there you are, standing on the summit, looking around at the magnificent view and feeling elated by the whole experience.

Reaching orgasm is just like this. As our sexual arousal becomes stronger (climbs), we experience more and more intense feelings until, suddenly, there we are at the peak of the (arousal) hill, feeling wonderful as a wave of exquisite pleasure flows over us.

For those of you who prefer a more practical than sublime description, orgasm has also been likened to a sneeze. You know how it is: you start with the *aah, aah, aah* (getting closer and closer to the sneeze) and then finish with the *aaahchew*. And isn't it a nice feeling when you finally get to that last . . . *chew*? You're left feeling relaxed, released and somehow satisfied. So it is with orgasm.

ↄ

LET ME RETURN to my story of the arousal hill. Just as most mountains and hills have different terrain, so it is with our sexual arousal hill.

We can experience steep bits where our feelings climb sharply, flat parts (plateaus) where our sexual feelings even out, and dips (valleys) where they seem to quiet down a little. You need to know the varying terrain of your arousal hill in order to understand what happens when you get turned on.

To make things a little more interesting, the shape of your arousal hill can change from one sexual occasion to another. For example, on one day it may be very steep and, on another, it could be a gentle slope. But don't worry if you're unsure of what your arousal hill looks like. The Programs outlined in chapters 13 and 14 will give you a chance to learn this.

> **NOTE:** (for the less fit among us): Don't be put off by all this talk of climbing hills, valleys and plateaus; believe me, it takes far less energy than a walk up a real hill, and provides just as many health benefits! It may also be more fun.

## stages of sexual arousal |

I FIND IT helpful to think of our sexual arousal as going through different stages while it builds towards orgasm.

- **STAGE 1: willingness**

  We must want to climb the arousal hill. In other words, we must *want* to have feelings of sexual pleasure. And we must *want* to put ourselves in the situation where we could get turned on. With *willingness* we are ready to be sexually stimulated by our triggers. We're standing at the bottom of the arousal hill and thinking about how nice it would be to make the climb and see the view.

- **STAGE 2: sensual awareness**

  We become aware that something or someone is triggering our sexual and romantic feelings. We feel positive, enjoying and wanting the experience. Our attention begins to shift to our body. We feel ourselves soften and open up; we notice warm, pleasant sensations, the first tingling of sexual pleasure in our body. We've taken a few steps up the arousal hill and know there's a pleasant journey ahead if we want it—and the possibility of a beautiful view from the top.

There are many different ways in which this sensual awareness can be expressed. For example, one woman may experience the pleasure feelings in her body and spend a few moments enjoying them—but do nothing else. Another may be aware of a need to press her body against that of her partner. Still another may begin thinking sexy thoughts while touching herself, in order to build the feelings further.

## STAGE 3: sexual excitement

We find the pleasant, warm sensations becoming more intense. We feel a sharper sense of pleasure that we clearly recognize as "sexual" pleasure. It seems to center around our genitals and spreads to other parts of our body. A feeling of warmth radiates through our body. We are beginning to get turned on. We feel ourselves become emotionally and physically excited. All these sensations become stronger as we begin to get involved in sexual activity. Each of our senses become focused on what we're doing. We've started climbing our arousal hill.

## STAGE 4: the valleys and plateaus

Sexual feelings don't always head straight to the top of the arousal hill. Depending on our mood, the strength of the sexual triggers, what's happening around us, and so on, our arousal may increase in strength, decrease, or level out for a while. If sexual stimulation continues *and* we stay interested in what's happening, our sexual feelings will grow in intensity. Gradually our body gathers itself together for the buildup to orgasm. Just before the final climb to the top, our feelings may level out for a while, as if we're sitting on a rock to catch our breath before continuing our climb.

The leveling out of the plateaus and the ups and downs of the valleys may happen once or several times (or never, if we're particularly excited by the sexual situation, and our arousal continues to increase in intensity). The terrain of our arousal hill may differ on each occasion of sexual activity. We may sometimes experience a smooth climb when it's possible to stay really focused on the sexual situation. At other times, when nonsexual thoughts or events distract us, it will be a bumpier ascent.

- **STAGE 5: orgasm**

Our sexual pleasure starts to become more intense, growing stronger and stronger. We focus on the sensations felt in our genitals. We sense we're coming close to seeing the lovely view from the top. And then we feel a sudden surge of a wonderful warm syrupy feeling flowing through our body as we reach the summit and look over the edge. Our vulva, clitoris, and vagina (in fact, our whole pelvis) will throb, making the feelings of pleasure even more enjoyable. For a short while we sit on the top and let the waves of pleasure flow through our body. We are enjoying the view. This peak of our arousal is the orgasm.

- **STAGE 6: relaxation**

The orgasm leaves us with a warm, tingly feeling and a sense (at least for a while) of well being. Our feelings, thoughts and body quietly settle down again. Slowly, feeling relaxed and at peace, we amble back down the hill—until the next time we decide to take the climb.

Some women like to have one orgasm and then rest at the bottom of the hill until another sexual occasion. Some enjoy repeating the whole experience again soon after the first orgasm. They have wandered down to a plateau or valley bottom, sat for a while and then begun, once again, to climb to the top. Others have no set pattern, but will wait to see how they feel after a short breather. On some days they may wish to climb to the top of the hill again. On other days they may enjoy the feelings of peace that follow orgasm.

**Each woman will climb the arousal hill in her own way. There's no right or wrong way, just YOUR way.**

It all depends on your mood, the kind of person you are, the setting in which you're being sexual, your partner, how tired you are, the triggers available, what you've been taught about sexual feelings by your culture, your level of physical fitness and so on. *Hundreds* of factors can affect the way your sexual arousal builds. It might build quickly or slowly, steadily or in spurts. And this can be different each time you get turned on.

If many sexual triggers become involved, this will help you to feel strong and steady arousal, leading to satisfying orgasm. If few sexual triggers are involved, you may find the climb to orgasm slower and the climax less satisfying.

## orgasm |

NOW, LET'S LOOK a little more closely at what orgasm means. It also involves both physical and psychological changes.

### THE PHYSICAL CHANGES

As we get more and more aroused, all the physical changes I described earlier continue. High levels of arousal also lead to the outer labia opening out and the vaginal entrance becoming more flexible. These changes allow you to more easily let a penis, finger, vibrator, or dildo be placed in your vagina.

If you took a look at yourself during orgasm, you'd notice that your breasts, chest, and neck area have become a deeper pink.

Your muscles will also have become more tense, and breathing and heart rate will have increased. Sometimes breathing too fast and lightly can lead to *hyperventilation*. If this happens, you may feel dizzy, and your hands, feet, and mouth may become numb. Don't worry. This is a temporary reaction and can easily be changed by breathing more deeply and slowly.

During high sexual arousal, the amount of blood flowing into the pelvic area increases. This makes all areas of the clitoris swell as much as possible and become even more sensitive.

When the blood vessels of the clitoris are filled, the valves in the arteries and veins close. This stops the blood from flowing out of the clitoris and creates a feeling of pressure or fullness in the pelvic area.

Feeling "bloated" or "tight" are other words used to describe this feeling. We call this **vasocongestion** or **pelvic congestion.**

At this time, you will want a constant and steady touch to your
clitoris.

---

I get so furious when my partner doesn't do this.
Just as I start to build up to a climax, he changes
the rhythm or touches me in a different place.
I tell him to keep going, but he laughs and thinks
I should just enjoy whatever he does.

---

You *would* feel mad about that. A steady rhythmical touch pushes
our sexual system to higher and higher levels of excitement. Anything
else seems a distraction and can be *most* frustrating.

If your arousal keeps building in the way I've described, the tension increases until there is a sudden peaking of pleasure. It's as if
your body can't go any further. You've reached a point of overload,
just like an electrical circuit board that blows a fuse. All your sexual
tension seems to explode, and the pelvic muscles begin to pulse in
a set of quick, rhythmical contractions. THIS IS ORGASM.

At orgasm, the layers of muscle in our pelvic area tighten in uni-
son. The outer layers contract in a rhythmical way, squeezing the
swollen and sensitive tissues of the clitoris. The deeper muscles also
move rhythmically, pressing against the inner clitoral tissue and tightening the vagina, bladder, and uterus. We feel a throbbing in our
pelvis that is very pleasurable.

Women can be very different in the way they feel these muscle
contractions. Some experience them as waves of throbbing that
seem to flow through the entire body, filling it with sexual pleasure.
Some find their legs start to shake or jerk. Others feel just a slight
vibration.

All this happens automatically as part of orgasm. But during or just
after orgasm, if you try tightening these muscles yourself in a steady
rhythm, it's possible to increase and continue the pleasurable feelings.

At orgasm, there is also an ejaculation of fluid from the paraurethral glands. With the help of muscle contractions, this will leave

the body through the urethra. However, it won't be obvious if the amount of ejaculation is very small.

With orgasm, the valves in the arteries and veins open, the blood is then released and flows back to other parts of the body. Our muscles relax again, and breathing and heart rates become normal.

If you don't orgasm but have felt quite sexually aroused, you may find yourself left with pelvic congestion. You'll feel this as an ache in the lower pelvis and clitoris caused by the pressure of blood that isn't able to be released. Don't worry. Everything should go back to normal after a time (if, of course, there are no more sexual triggers to set you off again).

## orgasm

### THE PSYCHOLOGICAL CHANGES

Orgasms are also experienced in an emotional and mental (psychological) way. Emotionally, we may feel fulfilled, satisfied, calm, relaxed, frustrated, resentful, overwhelmed, romantic, loved, unloved, childlike, and so on, depending on what the sexual experience means to us.

We all have attitudes towards orgasms, even if these ideas aren't something we stop and think about. Below are some examples of how an orgasm is viewed by some women:

- a way of showing love
- being a successful lover
- being a "real" woman
- the result of being in a trusting relationship
- a sign of being confident or close with a partner
- giving in to sexual feelings
- being vulnerable
- expressing an urge
- a gift, to give or receive
- a reward
- being fulfilled
- losing control of feelings

In other words, orgasms mean different things to different people. And, how we feel and think about orgasms (or having orgasms) plays a big part in the sexual experience we actually have. In fact, it's often the *emotions* and *thoughts* we have about orgasms that increase or decrease our level of sexual pleasure.

For example, you may see having an orgasm as being *a way of showing your love*. If you're with a partner you care about, this belief will help you to open up and let your arousal grow stronger, until you orgasm. But if your attitude is that orgasms are a way of losing control, then you may close up and stop yourself from getting close to orgasm.

I suppose it's a bit like baking a cake. If you put in fresh, healthy ingredients (healthy or positive thoughts and emotions as well as a healthy body), blend them really well, and allow the mixture to cook without interruption, you'll end up with a tasty cake (an orgasm).

---

Oh dear! I'm beginning to see the problem.
My ingredients are made up of bad attitudes and
stressed emotions, so the mixture is awfully lumpy
before I start. And then there are just too many
interruptions in my life to allow anything nice to cook.

---

You have it! But, you're not alone. There are many women, of all ages, who've been using the same recipe. Hopefully, this book will offer some new cooking tips.

## differences in feelings of orgasm |

THERE IS NO *right* way to feel an orgasm. I'm sure it won't surprise you to read this. The message I've given throughout this chapter has been that women can be quite different in the ways they express their sexual pleasure. Let's look at some of the different ways in which women experience orgasms.

Did you know, for example, that it's possible to have an orgasm *without being touched at all?* It usually happens when we're asleep and dreaming about something sexy. Our dreams (thoughts and emotions) act like a sexual trigger, getting our body so aroused that we experi-ence orgasm. Often we wake up just at this delicious moment.

You may also be able to orgasm this way when awake by think-ing about an exciting sexual fantasy. Don't worry if you can't. The look-no-hands approach seems easier when we're asleep and not so easily distracted.

I've mentioned before that some women ejaculate when having an orgasm. I want to touch on this again to remind you that it's a nat-ural and common way in which women experience their orgasm. One study found that four out of ten women ejaculated.[6] That's nearly half of the women questioned!

Ejaculation can happen whether you prefer clitoral or vaginal touching. However, most women who ejaculate also seem to have a very sensitive G-spot. Some women don't even have to wait for orgasm to ejaculate, but can do so when highly aroused.

Another way of experiencing orgasm is found in women with spinal-cord injuries. Because of this injury, the nerves of the spinal cord between the clitoris and brain are cut. This stops sexual mes-sages passing between the brain and the genitals. Yet, some of these women can feel orgasm when their vagina and cervix are firmly stroked in a rhythmical way. It's thought that sexual messages are sent from these areas to the brain and back again by the intestinal nerve network, in particular, the vagus nerve.[7]

And, interestingly, women with spinal cord damage often find that new areas of their body become super-sensitive to touch and give enjoyable feelings of sexual pleasure.

It's amazing, don't you think, how varied we are when it comes to sexual arousal and orgasms?

Orgasms can not only vary from woman to woman, but also from one sexual moment to the next. They can be:

- intense
- short
- mellow
- soft
- unexpected
- lingering
- quiet

- dramatic
- rippling
- fluttering
- bittersweet
- explosive
- and just about anything else you can think of

Some women find that the orgasm they experience from clitoral stimulation is different from the one felt when their vagina and G-spot are touched. Other women feel no difference.

The quality of orgasms can also change as a woman's body changes physically. As women get older, they may find their orgasms becoming less intense or not lasting as long as they used to. Some women find that the peak of their sexual pleasure is lower than it used to be— as if the top of the arousal hill is not quite as high as before. Other changes often found to occur with age are: the need for more time to get highly aroused and to orgasm; and the need to press harder to get a sexual reaction in the clitoris.

These alterations are caused by physical changes due to aging: shrinking of the clitoris; less swelling of the erectile tissue; slower nerve reactions; less sensitivity of the clitoral tissue; less muscle tension. Some of these changes are due to low levels of hormones (estrogen and androgens).

However, some older women find their orgasms becoming more intense at menopause. And many older women say they feel very satisfied sexually, despite the physical changes taking place in their bodies.

Pregnant women can also find their orgasms changing, as a result of hormonal changes. In addition, as we'll see in later chapters, some medical conditions can have the effect of altering the feelings of arousal and orgasm.

❧

HOPEFULLY MY MESSAGE is loud and clear: *there is no right way to feel an orgasm*. In fact, there are probably more ways of experiencing a climax than there are cake recipes. It all depends on your mood, levels of tiredness, involvement in the situation, partner's lovemaking ability,

time in the menstrual cycle, fitness levels, and a whole range of factors that can affect the way we think, feel, and act.

# orgasm difficulties |

NOW LET ME turn to the topic dear to your heart: orgasm
difficulties. Did you realize, as I described the stages of arousal, that
your problem is not with the first two stages (unless you're now so
frustrated by being unable to orgasm that you're no longer *willing* to
get started). It's the next three stages that are difficult.

Orgasm difficulties can be related back to either:

- **Being unable to continue up the arousal hill** because your feelings of pleasure sure seem to . . .
  - disappear
  - simmer on low heat, but never get to boiling point
  - go up and down the valleys
  - get stuck on a plateau

- **Being able to climb the arousal hill, but not being able to climax.**
  You . . .
  - get sooo close to orgasm, but can't quite reach the climax
    point
  - never get aroused high enough to feel that orgasm is just
    over the next rise

- **Being unable to have the kind of orgasm you used to have.** Your
  orgasm . . .
  - is barely noticeable
  - is over in an instant
  - is happening less and less
  - doesn't reach the peak of intensity it used to

In simple terms, your journey up the arousal hill is disturbed, and
you cannot reach the top.

## two paths to sexual feelings |

YOU'RE PROBABLY ITCHING for me to talk about what stops you from running back up the valleys, leaping off those plateaus, and racing up the arousal hill. Before I do this, however, there are a couple more things you need to know about getting turned on.

In simple terms, my previous comments boil down to the fact that there are two main ways in which you become aroused. The *first* is by having your body touched directly (either by yourself or a partner). Many parts of the body have the potential to turn us on sexually, although breasts, clitoris, and vagina are special favorites for most women.

The *second* way we get turned on is by reacting to sexual triggers with positive sexy thoughts (and feeling positive emotions that go with these thoughts). Because our nerves directly connect our brain and our genitals, whatever thoughts we have in our brain will affect our sexual arousal.

It's important to know that some thoughts have the effect of turning us *on*, while others do just the *opposite*. Imagine a switch in your brain that you can use to turn yourself on or off sexually. Here are some examples of how you can turn the switch on:

- ✓ fantasize: shut your eyes and picture a sexy scene
- ✓ daydream about someone you find sexy
- ✓ read romantic novels
- ✓ remember a time of lovemaking you really enjoyed
- ✓ think about music that reminds you of a very romantic or sexy movie

Thinking like this, you'll send positive "turn on" messages down to your clitoris. The result will be nice sexy feelings.

Now, here are some examples of how you can use the arousal switch to turn yourself off sexually:

- ✗ think of sex as bad
- ✗ feel guilty about enjoying yourself
- ✗ worry about a chore that isn't finished

✗ think over and over about not being able to orgasm
✗ concentrate hard on pleasing your partner, while thinking your sexual feelings are not as important

With negative thoughts like these, you'll soon find yourself without any sexy feelings.

---

Hey, are you telling me that my brain is really a sex organ?

---

I sure am. Probably the most important sex organ you have. As I describe the causes of orgasm difficulties in the next few chapters, you'll see that most of them involve some kind of negative thinking that acts as a turn-off to sexual feelings.

This is how it works. When we're thinking negatively, we become lost in our thoughts, rather than in the sexual situation. We're thinking *about* what we're doing (and why we're not happy with it), rather than simply *feeling* the pleasure of sexual reactions.

**The result is that we become a spectator at our own sexual "event."**

And it's not only negative thoughts that can affect us in this way. Emotions can also stop us from relaxing and enjoying our sexual pleasure. Anxiety and fear are examples of emotions that can have this affect. So, too, are stress, depression, anger, and resentment.

So, dear reader, negative thoughts and emotions are likely to be playing a part in keeping you on the plateaus and valleys of sexual arousal. For some of you, this will be a *large* part. In the next three chapters, I'll show you how this can happen.

## the turn-on, turn-off tug of war |

BUT, THERE'S MORE! What do you think happens when your clitoris, breasts, and other sexually sensitive parts of your body are being touched directly, either by yourself or someone else, and at the same time you're thinking negative "turn-off" thoughts?

*A huge tug of war goes on inside you*, that's what!

You set off a conflict between the source of arousal that is turn-ing you on (for example, your partner's touch) and the source that is turning you off (for example, a negative thought you have about your body shape).

---

So, this is why sex feels like such HARD work?
One cancels out the other.
No wonder I feel like I've run a marathon!

---

You're absolutely right. As you become sexually aroused, the turn-off messages work hard to stop any pleasure you're feeling. It really is a battle. You may get a little, or even moderately aroused, but it won't be enough to go on to orgasm.

Any time you think or feel negatively about sex or your sexual reactions, remember that you're doing a great job of dampening down your sexual feelings. And you're doing it all by yourself (even if someone in your past was responsible for teaching you to think or feel so negatively).

It can also work the other way. Some physical or medical condi-tions can dampen down your feelings of pleasure. They may, for example, stop the clitoris from filling with enough blood to give intense sexual feelings. Or your muscles may be unable to contract strongly enough. In these situations, you may be thinking in a very positive way, but it's your body that is dampening down your feelings.

Of course, if you're thinking negatively and your body isn't responding fully, then you don't have a tug of war at all—just a dou-ble dose of turn-off.

## causes of orgasm difficulties |

IN THE NEXT three chapters we're going to look at why you experience this sexual tug of war. Not surprisingly, the two pathways of sexual arousal can both be affected by relationship, fam-ily, personality, physical, and environmental circumstances. I find it helpful to break these elements down into three types of causes:

- **Causes that *lead* us to have problems (often occurring when we're girls or young women).**

  For example, being taught negative attitudes about sexual arousal. So many women have been told, *Don't let someone touch you down there until you're married or in a good relationship.* This often results in anxiety about sexuality that makes it hard to fully enjoy sexual pleasure.

- **Causes that seem to *start off* our orgasm difficulties.**

  For example, pressure from a partner to orgasm when you're just learning about sexual arousal and lack confidence as to what to do. Another example is starting to take anti-depression medication, which can dampen sexual arousal.

- **Causes that *keep* the problem going.**

  For example, being unable to relax during sex because of concern about a sick baby. Another example is worrying that you're not going to be able to orgasm.

As you read through the next three chapters, I'll be helping you to identify the causes behind your orgasm difficulty. Some of these will be causes which have made it likely that you would have problems experiencing orgasm, some will have actually triggered your orgasm difficulty, and some will be keeping it going.

**And, another thing:** after each cause is outlined, I'll ask you to rate how much you've been influenced by each one. It takes only ten seconds to complete them, so take the time to fill out the rating scales. In chapter 7 we'll bring all your ratings together, and this will show you what areas need changing.

⌒

NOW, LET'S BEGIN with those women who never or rarely have orgasms.

# 4

# why me?
## women who never or only occasionally have orgasms

**M**ANY WOMEN who have never or only occasionally experienced orgasms often ask,

> *Why me? How come I'm so different from all those other women who orgasm easily?*

The truth is that the only difference likely to exist between you and women who do orgasm is the *level of arousal you reach during sexual activity.* As I explained in chapter 3, you can get turned on, just as women who orgasm do, but your arousal level isn't high enough to orgasm. It probably feels as if your arousal gets stuck at a certain point and can't go further.

---

Absolutely, there are times when I've been getting turned on, and then I seem to hit a brick wall and the feelings just fade away.

---

...And the longer you keep trying to get more aroused, the more sensitive your clitoris will get.

_____

And then I can't stand to be touched any more.

_____

Exactly. Which means you have *no* chance of increasing your arousal.

I'm sure you know all this, so why don't we move on to something more interesting?—like how to change this situation.

But first, take a look at the following finding from a study done in the mid-1990s.[8] The study interviewed American women and found that:

> • 10% of the women studied rarely or never had an orgasm (in the previous twelve months)

This means that for every twenty women you meet, two will have exactly the same kind of orgasm difficulty you do. And a few more are likely to have different types of orgasm difficulties (but I'll talk about these in chapters 5 and 6). Did you think you'd be the only woman reading this chapter? I guess not!

It's now time for you to learn how to turn *some* arousal into *more* arousal (and orgasm). The first step is to *understand* why you can't get highly aroused and orgasm.

**The first steps to changing any behavior involve being AWARE of what you're doing and knowing WHY you do what you do.**

For those women who never or only occasionally orgasm, there are several possible reasons why this might happen. I've listed them in the box following:

## causes of orgasm difficulties:
### women who never or only occasionally orgasm

**Cause #1:** Being a busy person
**Cause #2:** Being goal-focused
**Cause #3:** Needing to stay in control of emotions
**Cause #4:** Lacking enough information about sexual arousal
**Cause #5:** Unable to communicate sexual needs
**Cause #6:** Not enough time to become highly aroused
**Cause #7:** Some fantasies can affect arousal
**Cause #8:** Feeling guilty about enjoying yourself
**Cause #9:** Feeling guilty because of childhood sex
**Cause #10:** Past sexual abuse
**Cause #11:** Long-term use of some medications
**Cause #12:** Physical conditions

Read through the description of each cause below, decide how much you believe it has affected you, and then mark the rating scale. It only takes a second to do this, so take the time. Later, as I've mentioned, we'll put all the ratings together, and you'll be able to see more clearly just why it is that you have difficulties with orgasm.

# CAUSE #1: |
## being a busy person

NO DOUBT YOU'RE scratching your head, wondering what on earth being busy has to do with orgasm. A great deal, as you will see.

Most women are very busy. They're usually working all day, whether at home or in the paid workforce. Then, at night there's the meal to get, children to look after, extra work or studies to do, a partner to relate to, parents and friends to call, housework to get done, exercise to fit in . . . and so it goes.

Weekends aren't much different; just add sport, socializing, and gardening to the list. There's little time for quiet relaxing.

---

Listen, I'd give a week's wages to be able to have time for myself, but I have so much to do there's no time to even SPELL the word relax.

---

Yes, I know. That's how it is for most women these days. Now, let me tell you how this relates to sexual arousal.

Think for a moment about what happens when you finally get to squeeze sex into your weekly routine. Do you find it hard to switch off from whatever you were doing half an hour before? Probably. I can picture it now. There you are, wanting to relax enough to really let your sexual feelings blossom, but it just doesn't happen. You're either wound up or exhausted, and sexual feelings simply can't *compete*.

When this happens we often become impatient. Getting aroused requires too much effort and time. We just want to forget about the orgasm. Besides, there are too many other things to do (or sleep seems *much* more attractive).

You can see the problem, can't you? There's simply not enough time or the right attitude for you to gradually move through the stages of arousal.

Sometimes, it's a partner who gets impatient. He or she may already feel quite aroused and want to rush into sex. The problem is, you haven't had time to slowly unwind from the day. You're simply not ready to let go and get highly aroused. Which probably makes you cranky and even less able to relax.

Sexual feelings are a bit like a tropical flower. They need tender loving care if they're to blossom. Being relaxed (and awake) is an important ingredient in our sexual blossoming.

Think about my comments and how they fit your situation. Now take a few moments to fill in the rating scale below. Place an X next to the answers that seem to fit you.

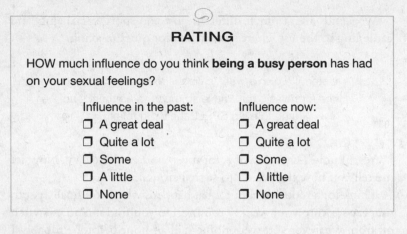

**RATING**

HOW much influence do you think **being a busy person** has had on your sexual feelings?

| Influence in the past: | Influence now: |
| --- | --- |
| ❏ A great deal | ❏ A great deal |
| ❏ Quite a lot | ❏ Quite a lot |
| ❏ Some | ❏ Some |
| ❏ A little | ❏ A little |
| ❏ None | ❏ None |

# CAUSE #2:
## being goal-focused

SOME PEOPLE LIKE to be productive. In fact they like it so much that everything they do is governed by a goal they hope to achieve. See if any of the following comments remind you of *you:*

*Today I'm going to make sure I get the garden weeded*
(And you don't stop until it's done).

*This morning I'm going to clear my in-tray*
(And you don't stop until it's done).

*Now that I have some spare time, I plan to clean out that cupboard*
(And you don't stop until it's done).

Women who think like this set goals for themselves. Then they put a lot of effort into what needs to be done to meet those goals. Now, let me be clear: I'm not against being productive or goal-focused. It's very satisfying to set yourself a goal and to reach it.

Problems arise, though, when reaching a particular goal or completing a task is the *only* thing that takes your attention.

Are you one of these women? Do you become so focused on reaching your goal that everything else is ignored? Do you forget to enjoy yourself as you work towards your goal? Is it hard to stop what you're doing even if you become too tired to finish the task? Do you keep doing chores while talking to a friend on the phone?

If the answer is yes, then it's time to face up to the fact that you're probably *too* goal-focused.

Does being too goal-focused stop you from enjoying sex and having orgasms? You bet it does. Sex can't be treated like another task, with orgasm as the goal. In fact, setting up orgasm as a goal to be achieved is a sure way to make certain you *don't* have one.

---

But I usually get a lot done when I set goals for myself. Why can't I do the same with orgasms?

---

Good question. The answer is that sexual arousal gets stronger by *feeling* the emotions and physical reactions that occur during sex. The minute you start *thinking about* having an orgasm, and tensing yourself to *work* at it, you'll be distracted from the emotions and reactions. And then you can just wave your orgasm goodbye.

It doesn't matter if you think something positive, such as,

*I'm determined to have an orgasm this time,*

or something hopeful, such as,

*Please God, let me do it this time,*

or something despairing, such as,

*It's hopeless, I know I won't get there this time,*

the result will still be the same. Thoughts like these focus attention on what you want to *produce* from sex. You are *thinking about* your goal. Thinking hard. Thinking negatively. Judging whether you're good enough. Pressuring yourself to reach the elusive goal.

Are you getting the picture? You've become a *spectator*, looking at, and judging, your own sexual performance. *How am I doing? Will I make it? What is my partner thinking of me?*

What chance do you have of really getting turned on? Very little, I can tell you.

**You're so busy being a spectator that you've stopped being a participant.**

As if this isn't enough, some women who are goal-focused are also never satisfied with anything they achieve. Being *perfectionists*, they're only too ready to criticize their behavior. With this approach, there's probably little chance they'll being able to relax and become absorbed in the sexual moment as a participant, rather than a very judgmental spectator.

Being a perfectionist sets up a fear of failing. And this, in turn, creates feelings of anxiety. The problem is that during sex, anxiety competes with feelings of arousal. If the anxiety is strong enough, it will overtake the sexual arousal and "switch" it off. The closer you get to the goal (orgasm) that you fear you won't achieve, the stronger the anxiety and the more likely you are to switch off your sexual feelings.

I often describe sex as *adult play*. Think about how young children play. Have you noticed how absorbed they are in what they're doing at any moment? Yes, they're totally focused on what they're doing. But it's not a task to be completed. There's no pressure to reach a goal. They're simply lost in the play, with no thought *about* what they're doing.

As adults, we often forget how to be this absorbed. Instead of *playing* sexually in a relaxed, spontaneous and enjoyable way, we set up a kind of sweatshop where we *work hard* at achieving our *goal* of orgasm.

The idea that you have to somehow "work at an orgasm" will actually prevent your having one. Firstly, you are placing *soooo* much pressure on yourself that you can never be relaxed enough to allow arousal to build. Secondly (and more importantly), your emphasis on the goal of orgasm means that your attention is on the *future* (having an orgasm) rather than on the *present* (your emotions and body sensations).

Take a few moments to consider my comments, and then rate yourself as honestly as you can.

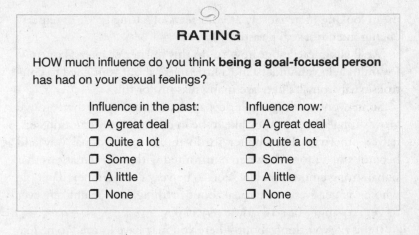

**RATING**

HOW much influence do you think **being a goal-focused person** has had on your sexual feelings?

| Influence in the past: | Influence now: |
|---|---|
| ❒ A great deal | ❒ A great deal |
| ❒ Quite a lot | ❒ Quite a lot |
| ❒ Some | ❒ Some |
| ❒ A little | ❒ A little |
| ❒ None | ❒ None |

## CAUSE #3:
### needing to stay in control of emotions

ONE OF THE most common reasons women never or only rarely experience orgasm is that they have difficulty letting go of control over their sexual feelings.

In the sexual setting they can usually let themselves feel sexually aroused, but only up to a certain point. When their sexual feelings begin to build, they become uncomfortable and try to take control. They may do this deliberately or be completely unaware of their reactions. Their sexual arousal gets to a plateau and either stays there or fades away (going down into a valley or returning to the bottom of the arousal hill again).

Does this seem to describe you? If so, then I need to warn you that it's *impossible* to orgasm without letting go of the controls for a brief moment. Did you know that at the moment of orgasm, our body sensations and emotions are actually out of control? It's true. It may be a short or long moment. But, like a sneeze, it's a moment when you must let go and allow the feelings and sensations to flow through you.

So, dear reader, you are faced with an interesting dilemma. Either stay in control and feel more at ease (but not orgasmic), *or* learn to overcome your discomfort with uncontrolled feelings. This could mean looking more closely at your fears of letting go or of experiencing intense sexual pleasure.

We'll talk more about how to do this in later chapters. For now, I want to help you understand a little more about your need to control sexual arousal. There are many reasons for this.

Some women, for example, feel anxious about letting their arousal grow stronger because they like to be in control of *any* emotion, sexual or otherwise. They prefer to do things in a rational way and become uncomfortable when confronted with body sensations that signal strong emotions. They tend to be very even-tempered people who never get overly emotional about anything. They're unlikely ever to get *very* angry or *very* sad or *very* happy.

If this fits you, think about where you may have learned to be like this. Perhaps you came from a family or culture in which emotions were suppressed. This would have given you little experience of expressing a range of emotions.

Perhaps it was quite the opposite situation. Strong emotions, such as parental anger, can lead a little girl to control her reactions in order to avoid being the target of that anger.

Whatever your background, keep in mind that sexual arousal is no different from other emotions. So, how you cope with emotions generally may be the key to what happens when your feelings of sexual pleasure begin to build.

It's not only our upbringing that can teach us to control emotions. Painful experiences occurring at any time in our life can do the same. Sometimes these experiences can leave us with emotions that are stressful. Grief, anger, and hurt are examples of this. Often we bury them inside, trying to ignore them, for fear they'll pop up again.

The problem is, these buried emotions can still interfere with having an orgasm. How is that? Remember, at orgasm we have to let go for a few moments. So, at this time, it's possible for any emotions being held tightly inside to come to the surface. Somehow, we sense this—and hold back our arousal.

Perhaps you've heard that women sometimes cry at the point of orgasm. Although some cry for joy, many cry because they feel sad or hurt inside. At orgasm, they're unable to control this sadness or hurt, and it surfaces with the sexual climax. Funnily, these women usually feel a great sense of release and peace when this happens.

Having sex with a partner can often make things worse for women who control emotions. Why? Because the thought of showing emotions in front of another person will increase their feelings of awkwardness and embarrassment. Perhaps they never cry, get angry or dissolve into laughter with others. The thought of doing so may fill them with horror.

Sometimes it's the fear of being emotionally vulnerable that worries women. They believe that showing or letting out feelings will put them at risk of getting hurt.

On the other hand, there are women who have trouble letting go of control over sexual feelings because the whole idea of being "passionate" scares them. They worry about becoming a "wild woman." They feel nervous about being less inhibited in front of another. They worry about the noises or movements they could make as they become highly aroused.

-------

*Well, yes, I've always worried that when I have an orgasm, I'm going to look horrible. I know this is at the back of my mind during sex, so I guess it's affecting me.*

-------

You're probably right there. Some women do worry about what they look like to their partner. They're so concerned about presenting well that it's impossible to let themselves go and enjoy sexual pleasure. I'll bet, though, your partner is too preoccupied with making love to *you* to be noticing the look on your face.

**The truth is, we generally don't look much different during orgasm than when we're having a good laugh about something.**

By the way, did you know that partners usually find the sounds and movements of orgasm quite a turn-on?

If you're a young teenage girl who's started to feel sexual arousal only recently, you may be aware of *deliberately* holding back when you become too aroused. Perhaps you're afraid of getting carried away with your sexual feelings and ending up pregnant. Perhaps you're feeling guilty because your parents wouldn't like you behaving sexually (either on your own or with someone else).

Then again, maybe you're not sure what's happening when you experience a surge of sexual arousal. There are many women, young and old, who have this reaction. They feel anxious about where the growing sexual pleasure will take them. They're worried they'll urinate or explode or have something terrible happen (although they can't really say what this might be!). So, they tighten up physically and emotionally, and the result is that their sexual feelings build so far and no further. It's as if they're frightened of what they might see at the top of the hill—and therefore stop climbing.

Unfortunately, many women are discouraged from exploring their feelings of sexual pleasure by the negative messages parents and others have given them. Instead of learning that sexual arousal is pleasurable and fun, they've been told it's dangerous, naughty, revealing, selfish and unproductive (just to mention a few).

So, when these women begin to enjoy feelings of sexual arousal, they get scared, fearing some kind of punishment for going any further. There's not much chance, then, of feeling *high* sexual arousal, let alone enjoying an orgasm.

Now take a look at what happens when you start to get turned on. See if it goes something like this: *Get aroused. Stop. Get aroused. Stop. Get aroused. Stop.* This is how it is for many women who control their emotions. And after a while, this pattern will happen without thinking about it. You may feel as if every time you get *too* aroused, there's now an automatic switch which says, *Okay, that's enough, it's time to stop.*

---

Yes, that's me exactly. Just when I think I'm relaxed
and ready to feel more aroused, my feelings just
click off, without a moment's warning. It's absolutely
frustrating.

---

And difficult to stop! After several years of letting yourself get aroused so far and no further, your sexual feelings will become *conditioned* to turn off at a certain point. The longer you've been switching off in this way, the more automatic the turn-off will be.

However, it's also likely that the negative thought that started all this in the first place is still lurking deep in your brain. You know, the thought that goes something like: *it could be uncomfortable or embarrassing for me if I let myself get more turned on. I could get into trouble.* Unconscious thoughts like this can dampen sexual feelings just as much as thoughts you're fully aware of.

Since negative thoughts lead to negative emotions, the next step will be that you begin to feel rather anxious and tense. Then you certainly won't be feeling much sexual pleasure.

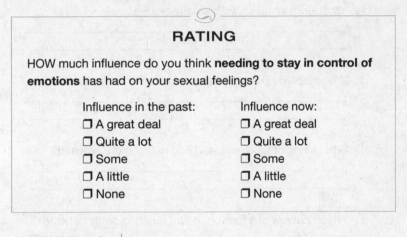

### RATING

HOW much influence do you think **needing to stay in control of emotions** has had on your sexual feelings?

| Influence in the past: | Influence now: |
| --- | --- |
| ❏ A great deal | ❏ A great deal |
| ❏ Quite a lot | ❏ Quite a lot |
| ❏ Some | ❏ Some |
| ❏ A little | ❏ A little |
| ❏ None | ❏ None |

## CAUSE #4:
### lacking enough information about sexual arousal

SOMETIMES IT'S A lack of information that makes it difficult to have orgasms. Many women, for example, have never heard of the different stages of sexual arousal. So when they experience their sexual feelings starting to level out at a plateau or sink into a valley, they think, *Oh no, I'm losing the feelings (again)* and then just stop all sexual activity.

If they'd known that it's perfectly natural for their sexual arousal to go up and down like this, they might have relaxed and enjoyed the moment until their arousal began to build towards a climax.

Unfortunately, women often lack information about what arousal is and how it changes through the different stages.

And another thing: many women don't know enough about their bodies, especially the clitoris. They may not understand its importance or the differences in sensitivity between the clitoris and the vagina. They may want to orgasm during intercourse and not be aware of how the clitoris plays a part in this happening. They may know little about how they need to be touched in order to keep their arousal building.

Let's see what you know about yourself. Try the following quiz:

# touch quiz

1. What *kinds* of touch will sexually arouse you?

   _____

   _____

2. *Where* do you like to be touched in order to get aroused?

   _____

   _____

3. What kinds of touch will lead you to feel *more* aroused?

   _____

   _____

4. Which is more of a turn-on, being touched softly or being touched firmly?

   _____

   _____

5. How does the type of touch you enjoy *change* as you get more aroused?

   _____

   _____

6. Do you need a different kind of touch at different times in your menstrual cycle?

   _____

   _____

7. Do you need a different kind of touch for different moods?

_____

_____

8. What happens to your level of sexual arousal when your breasts and nipples are stroked?

_____

_____

9. Are there other parts of your body which, when touched, make you feel sexy?

_____

_____

10. Do you feel comfortable telling your partner how you like to be caressed?

_____

_____

Take a few moments to write down your answers.

Wait a minute, I thought my partner
was supposed to know all this stuff, not me.

And if he or she *doesn't* know how to touch you, then what happens? How are your sexual needs going to be met? Perhaps this has been your problem: you've been waiting until your partner somehow "figures it out." The question is, how long do you plan to wait? It could take forever!

No, dear reader. While our partners *do* need to know what turns us on, it shouldn't be up to them to "figure it out." That's *our* job. *We* need to know what turns us on, and I'm not referring here just to touch. We need to know how we react to *all* our sexual triggers.

**You are the only one who can truly be an expert on your own sexual arousal.**

So, it's up to you to learn about what sexually arouses you and particularly what makes you *more* aroused. Remember, to have an orgasm we have to let ourselves become *very* aroused. If you're not being touched the way you like (either by yourself or a partner), then the chances are you won't get to orgasm.

Unfortunately, many young (and some not so young) women believe that when they aren't touched in an arousing way by their partner, it's because the partner doesn't really love or care for them. Well, think again!

There are several reasons for partners not touching us in the way we like. The obvious one is that, despite all the caring in the world, they simply don't know what we like (and either can't get the information from us or are afraid to ask).

Then again, a partner might find a particular touch a real turnon and so touch you in the same way, thinking it will work for you, too. Of course, it may be quite different from the kind of touch you like, leaving you feeling annoyed rather than turned on.

Before you blame your partner, then, it would be more helpful to accept that it's up to you to take responsibility for educating your partner as to how you like to be touched.

---

But I don't think I've stopped to notice
what I like and don't like.

---

You're not alone, believe me! Unfortunately, women aren't encouraged to explore their own bodies. Negative messages about our bodies come from all directions: parents, society, the church, and so on. This is a great pity because it stops women from becoming familiar with what their body needs to get turned on.

Many women learn about their sexual reactions when they masturbate or touch themselves. This is a great way of finding out about yourself. Why? Because you can explore what turns you on without the presence of another person to worry about. Masturbation is private, and you can concentrate just on yourself. Of course, it *is*

possible to learn with a sensitive partner who has a good understanding of women's sexuality. (But I guess this didn't happen, or you
wouldn't need to read my book.)

If you haven't masturbated, then you may not have given yourself
the chance to learn how to become fully aroused. Of course, if you've
tried masturbating half-heartedly, as many women do, then your heart
probably wasn't in it and you *definitely* wouldn't have given your
arousal a chance to develop.

---

But my mother, bless her religious soul, told me girls
shouldn't do THAT—you know, touch themselves
THERE. Whenever I try it, I hear her voice in my ear,
and boy, do I feel . . . ah . . . uncomfortable!

---

Many women would say the same thing. And would your mother
have given your brothers the same message? Probably not. You know
what they say: *boys will be boys!* It's usually women who are made to
feel there's something wrong with touching themselves in order to feel
sexual pleasure.

Yet, the ability to experience sexual pleasure is a natural part of
being a human being. The way I see it, if you feel negative about your
sexual ability, you're really feeling negative about *yourself.*

---

## RATING

HOW much influence do you think **lacking enough information
about sexual arousal** has had on your sexual feelings?

| Influence in the past: | Influence now: |
|---|---|
| ❏ A great deal | ❏ A great deal |
| ❏ Quite a lot | ❏ Quite a lot |
| ❏ Some | ❏ Some |
| ❏ A little | ❏ A little |
| ❏ None | ❏ None |

# CAUSE #5: |
## unable to communicate sexual needs

SOME WOMEN KNOW exactly how they like to be touched in order to get aroused, but are afraid to tell a partner. They may be worried about being ridiculed or, worse still, ignored. They may be nervous about offending or threatening their partner in some way. They may feel embarrassed about sharing such personal information.

---

*Hey, what am I going to say? Down lower. No, over to the right a bit. Yes, now harder. Back the other way. It's not exactly romantic, is it?*

---

No, I guess it isn't. But then how romantic is it to have you lying there feeling resentful because you're not being touched in the right way? Your partner may be quite ignorant of how you like to be touched. He or she isn't a mind reader.

Remember, even being in a loving, committed relationship doesn't mean your partner instantly knows everything about you. This is a common belief among women.

There are a few other beliefs that stop women from communicating about their sexual needs. One of these is the idea that if your partner is male, he should be experienced and know it all, and if female, she should know what to do because she's also a woman. Then there's the belief that if you talk about sex, it stops the mystery and romance. Another view is that if you and your partner truly love each other, orgasm will happen easily.

Sorry to tell you, but these are *mistaken* beliefs. There is *no* truth in them. Sex is no different from other areas of your life. A partner can't know what type of food you feel like eating or what movie you'd like to see. He or she can guess, but that's all it is . . . a guess. Some days it may be a good guess. Other days it may be off the mark and you could end up with food or a movie you dislike.

It's the same with sex. If you don't talk about what you need to become sexually aroused, your attention will soon turn to what's turning you *off*. Any arousal you might have had will stop, and you'll be sitting on a plateau, twiddling your thumbs. Then, as quickly as you can say, *My lips are sealed,* your feelings will be heading down into a valley, with little chance of recovery.

It's not surprising, therefore, that women who are sexually assertive have orgasms more often than women who aren't able to say what they need sexually.[9]

Being assertive about our sexual needs isn't always easy. Young women, in particular, find it hard to ask for what they need sexually. They think it makes them sound too eager or pushy. Those who enjoy sex are sometimes labeled with horrible names such as slut, nympho, and whore, and this can be enough to make some of them hold back sexually. (By the way, have you noticed that men *don't* get called horrible names for enjoying their sexual feelings?)

---

### RATING

HOW much influence do you think **being unable to communicate sexual needs** has had on your sexual feelings?

| Influence in the past: | Influence now: |
| --- | --- |
| ❐ A great deal | ❐ A great deal |
| ❐ Quite a lot | ❐ Quite a lot |
| ❐ Some | ❐ Some |
| ❐ A little | ❐ A little |
| ❐ None | ❐ None |

---

# CAUSE #6:
## not enough time to become highly aroused

MOST WOMEN NEED a period of time to become sexually aroused. Do you know how much time you need? Many don't! Some even try to model themselves on men, who seem to get aroused more quickly and easily. Then they give up or think there's something wrong with them if they don't become aroused at the same pace.

Yet, women are different. They usually need *time* to become relaxed, feel safe and get into a sexual mood. They also need to be *willing* to stay long enough to get aroused.

Being *willing* is important. A woman often starts lovemaking with a low level of sexual arousal. This is especially true if she is inhibited about sex, has been in a relationship for some time, has a busy life taking her attention, or is not one to initiate sexual activity.

But if she's *willing* to stay in the sexual situation, and has a partner who is prepared to take the time to allow her to become aroused, and doesn't feel pressurized to have an orgasm, she will usually be pleasantly surprised by how aroused she does become.

---

I know you're right. I never have time to feel in the
mood before he starts to get really turned on. I'm
just unwinding from work and the kids—and he's
ready to climax!

---

I've heard many women say exactly the same thing: they don't get enough time to become highly aroused. Of course, you also need to be willing to let everything else go from your mind and to stay in the sexual situation for the time you need.

By the way, it's no different if you're touching yourself, get impatient and give up. You still need to give *yourself* enough time.

Perhaps you're quite happy to take more time to get aroused, but your partner wants to get into the swing of things more quickly. There's nothing wrong with this. Having sex with a partner means there'll be *two* different arousal patterns. It's quite possible that one of you will become more quickly aroused than the other.

However, your partner may not realize this difference in your arousal levels. Remember, once we get turned on, our attention becomes more and more focused on our own feelings of sexual pleasure. So, if your partner's highly aroused, he or she may assume you're also getting ready to orgasm—when you're not!

None of this will matter if you can both enjoy the orgasm of your partner first and then go on to building your arousal and enjoying your orgasm. For some strange reason, however, many heterosexual (male/female) couples stop sexual activity after the man has had his orgasm. Which means there's no time given for you to get more aroused. The result? No orgasm.

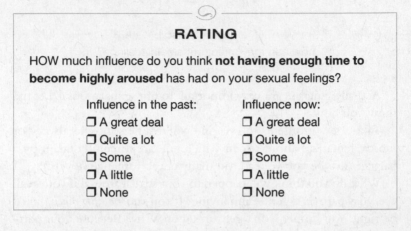

**RATING**

HOW much influence do you think **not having enough time to become highly aroused** has had on your sexual feelings?

Influence in the past:
❏ A great deal
❏ Quite a lot
❏ Some
❏ A little
❏ None

Influence now:
❏ A great deal
❏ Quite a lot
❏ Some
❏ A little
❏ None

# CAUSE #7:
## some fantasies can affect arousal

NOW, I WANT to talk about something quite different: the way fantasies can stop you from ever getting to orgasm. This may also be a cause of orgasm problems in women who orgasm at some times and not others (See chapter 6).

*Sexual fantasies* are stories or pictures we think about that have the ability to trigger our sexual arousal. Not everyone fantasizes—some people just can't seem to do this. But others find it very enjoyable.

We can imagine anything we like in our fantasies. You may picture a sexy scene with your partner or another person (this is much more common than you may think). You may recall a sexy memory that you now find particularly arousing, or imagine settings that you've never been in. Many women also like to fantasize about activities they wouldn't normally carry out in their sexual lives.

Some women worry about their fantasies, especially if they're about someone or something different. They get scared that fantasizing in this way will lead them to act out their thoughts in real life.

There is no need for this fear. Fantasies are just thoughts, your own private thoughts. They're only acted out if that's what you want. It's your choice.

---

Well, if fantasies are so private,
how can they affect our sexual feelings?

---

Actually, fantasies are very important to our sexual arousal. Let me show you how.

Take a few moments to imagine you're a person who always, or mostly, fantasizes about sex in which you are forcefully taken by a partner (maybe you've read too many cheap romance novels!).

What do you think will happen to your sexual arousal if your real, everyday partner is gentle and loving? If you said, *nothing much,* you'd be right! You simply won't get turned on. Why? Because your partner doesn't match the kind of lovemaking you always fantasize about.

The same thing would happen if you always fantasized about thin people, and your partner is big and cuddly. Or if you fantasize about women and your partner is a man. And so on.

When we stick to the *same* sexual picture, fantasy after fantasy, year after year, we become conditioned to *only* feeling sexually aroused by that fantasy. We teach our body that the trigger to sexual arousal is the fantasy we like so much.

However, this conditioning doesn't happen if we enjoy using several different fantasies and swap them around on a regular basis.

Interestingly, fantasies are the one exception where positive thoughts (which is what sexual fantasies usually are), rather than negative ones, cause orgasm difficulties.

---

## RATING

HOW much influence do you think **your fantasies** have had on your sexual feelings?

| Influence in the past: | Influence now: |
|---|---|
| ❒ A great deal | ❒ A great deal |
| ❒ Quite a lot | ❒ Quite a lot |
| ❒ Some | ❒ Some |
| ❒ A little | ❒ A little |
| ❒ None | ❒ None |

# CAUSE #8:
## feeling guilty about enjoying yourself

WOMEN OFTEN ADMIT to feeling guilty when it comes to sex. This usually means they believe they're doing something wrong and feel bad about it.

There are probably as many reasons women feel guilty during sex as there are stars in the sky. I've chosen to discuss just two, the two I think give the most problems for women who've never or only occasionally had an orgasm. In this section I'll concentrate on guilt about enjoying life. Cause #9 will look at guilt about childhood sexual feelings.

Let's begin by seeing what you're feeling guilty about. Try the Guilt Quiz below:

## guilt quiz

1. Do you feel guilty if you sit down to read a magazine when there are chores to be done?
   Yes ☐   No ☐

2. Do you feel guilty about going out to lunch when there are jobs to be done at home?
   Yes ☐   No ☐

3. Do you feel guilty if you're enjoying yourself at a party or social function?
   Yes ☐   No ☐

4. Does it feel selfish to be enjoying spending time with a partner when there are so many tasks you could get on with?
   Yes ☐   No ☐

Did you nod yes to any of these questions? Then it's no wonder that orgasm is difficult for you. If you feel guilty about enjoying yourself generally, you'll probably feel the same way about enjoying sex.

Guilt will lead you to hold back your feelings during sex. When your sexual arousal starts to build, you'll feel negative and worry about being lazy, selfish, irresponsible, or wasting time. The result will be that you switch off sexually.

Remember, sex is an adult version of play—it's about fun and pleasure. It's hard, though, to enjoy yourself when guilty feelings pop up. Let me give you an example of how guilt can affect sexual arousal.

I once counseled a woman who was eighteen years of age when she had her first sexual experience. In the middle of this experience, she had a pang of guilt. The thought, *It's not right to enjoy myself like this,* had popped into her head. Naturally, any sexual feelings instantly disappeared. Prior to the guilty thought, a picture of her mother (who, sadly, had died a year before) had flashed into her mind.

The phrase that came into her head, *It's not right to enjoy myself like this,* was learned in childhood when her mother was often ill. She and her brother had to be quiet and do many of the household chores. If they wanted to play, they'd feel guilty, since there was always something that needed doing. They also knew their mother was too sick to enjoy herself.

After her first sexual experience, this woman found that the guilty thought would come into her mind whenever she became highly aroused. She felt bad about enjoying herself too much and would use the thought to keep her arousal down to "acceptable" levels.

This is a good example of how being unable to enjoy yourself can lead to difficulty with orgasm.

## RATING

HOW much influence do you think **feeling guilty about enjoying yourself** has had on your sexual feelings?

| Influence in the past: | Influence now: |
| --- | --- |
| ❏ A great deal | ❏ A great deal |
| ❏ Quite a lot | ❏ Quite a lot |
| ❏ Some | ❏ Some |
| ❏ A little | ❏ A little |
| ❏ None | ❏ None |

# CAUSE #9:
## feeling guilty because of childhood sex

I'VE WORKED WITH many women who feel guilty as a result of what happened to them as a child when they had sexy feelings. This kind of guilt is often present in women who rarely or never orgasm. Unfortunately, it's too often overlooked as a cause of orgasm difficulties.

Let's first begin with some simple, but truthful observations. Children *do* feel sexual arousal and orgasms. As I mentioned in chapter 1, baby girls have been observed having an orgasm. And little girls are commonly seen to masturbate.

I also mentioned previously that children don't have the language or cultural knowledge to call what they're feeling *sexual*. They simply feel pleasurable feelings. They're enjoying themselves. When little girls touch themselves on the vulva and clitoris, it's usually because it gives them a nice feeling. Sometimes it's used as a form of comfort or to put themselves to sleep.

Unfortunately, this innocence can be shattered if an adult, such as a parent, reacts badly to seeing the child acting "sexually" (but remember the child doesn't understand this word). What follows usually sets the groundwork for adult guilt.

The adult verbally or physically attacks the child about her actions. In no time at all, the young girl has learned that her pleasurable feelings are wrong and bad. This teaching then becomes the basis for a negative attitude towards her own arousal.

The tragedy of this negative teaching soon becomes apparent when the little girl grows into an adult woman. As she starts to feel sexual pleasure, a little voice yells, *Stop being dirty, don't do that!*—or something similar. Deep in her subconscious she remembers the reactions of adults to her innocent child's behavior. So ingrained is the fear of this reaction that she switches off sexual feelings just as soon as sexual arousal begins to build. Without realizing it, she's trying to avoid being punished. Sexual feelings are shut down in order to escape the fear.

As if this weren't enough, as children and teenagers, women are often taught to feel guilty about sexual arousal, even if they haven't actually been punished for acting in a sexual way. The messages they hear are usually warnings about the terrible things that will happen if their sexual arousal gets out of control.

---

> How true! My mother used to say, Mary, be careful. We don't want you getting any diseases. Or, it was, "Behave yourself, there's plenty of time for sex later when you're older." I still did it, anyway, but I always felt as if my mother were watching me.

---

And that's a good way of learning to feel guilty. Unfortunately, this kind of warning translates for many into: *Don't let yourself get carried away with sexual passion.*

**In other words, don't become sexually aroused.**

Women learn it's fine to enjoy a cuddle and a kiss, but as soon as sexual arousal starts to build, the negative messages are recalled, the guilty feelings come to the surface and *sexual feelings are quickly shut down.* They learn to become aroused to a certain level (a safe level) and no further.

---

### RATING

HOW much influence do you think **feeling guilty because of childhood sex** has had on your sexual feelings?

| Influence in the past: | Influence now: |
|---|---|
| ❐ A great deal | ❐ A great deal |
| ❐ Quite a lot | ❐ Quite a lot |
| ❐ Some | ❐ Some |
| ❐ A little | ❐ A little |
| ❐ None | ❐ None |

---

## CAUSE #10:
### past sexual abuse

I WOULD DEFINE an event as sexually abusive if you're forced to do something sexual you don't want to do, if your sexual needs and preferences are ignored, and if you feel that others lack respect for your physical, mental and emotional safety. Abuse can involve physical as well as verbal attack.

Often sexual abuse stops women from feeling any kind of sexual arousal. The problem then is more likely to be *lack of sexual desire* rather than orgasm difficulties. However, some women find that while they can get turned on sexually, their arousal is never enough to orgasm.

Sexually abusive experiences, like any traumatic experience, can have a great impact on us. Our bodies learn to switch feelings off, to tense up in readiness of an attack, to be wary of trusting others, and to watch out for signs of sexual desire on the part of others.

This can make it difficult to let yourself go sexually. Even if you're in a loving relationship, it may still be difficult to relax and focus on your own sexual pleasure.

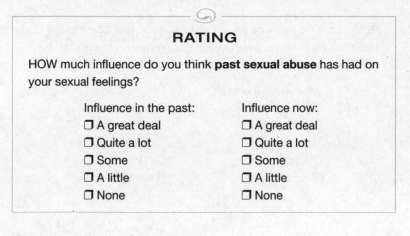

### RATING

HOW much influence do you think **past sexual abuse** has had on your sexual feelings?

| Influence in the past: | Influence now: |
|---|---|
| ❑ A great deal | ❑ A great deal |
| ❑ Quite a lot | ❑ Quite a lot |
| ❑ Some | ❑ Some |
| ❑ A little | ❑ A little |
| ❑ None | ❑ None |

## CAUSE #11:
### long-term use of some medications

ALTHOUGH SOME MEDICATIONS, such as antidepressants, tranquilizers, narcotics and beta adrenergic blockers, can dampen sexual arousal (See chapter 5), it's rare for this to be a cause of orgasm difficulties for a woman who never or only occasionally has an orgasm. However, I have sometimes talked with women who've been on antidepressants continuously since they were adolescents. In each case, I found that this medication was preventing them from experiencing an orgasm.

However, before you rush to throw away the bottle of pills (always talk to your doctor first), you should know that:

- Some antidepressants don't have this effect.
- Sexual side effects may only occur at certain dose levels.
- Some women are able to orgasm even when on medication that has a side effect of suppressing sexual arousal.

Take note, then, of the other causes of orgasm difficulties outlined in this chapter before assuming that medications could be affecting your ability to orgasm.

---

### RATING

HOW much influence do you think **long-term use of medications** has had on your sexual feelings? (Without a medical check, you can only guess at this.)

| Influence in the past: | Influence now: |
|---|---|
| ❒ A great deal | ❒ A great deal |
| ❒ Quite a lot | ❒ Quite a lot |
| ❒ Some | ❒ Some |
| ❒ A little | ❒ A little |
| ❒ None | ❒ None |

---

# CAUSE #12:
## physical conditions

IT'S RARE FOR there to be a physical condition that stops women from ever, or only occasionally, having an orgasm.

One example of such a condition is the presence of a clitoral skin adhesion (phimosis of the clitoris), a flap of skin that joins to the clitoris and may restrict sensitivity and movement.

Another possible physical cause is extreme weakness of the pelvic muscles (perhaps caused by a muscle-wasting disease) that makes it difficult to feel waves of muscle contraction at orgasm. Long-standing physical disabilities, such as paraplegia, can also make orgasm difficult.

Some forms of clitoridectomy, or the removal of parts of the clitoris (usually the glans and shaft) can make it difficult to reach high levels of arousal or may so weaken the feeling of orgasm that it is hardly noticeable. This practice is common in some areas of Africa, Asia, and the Middle East and is often used to prevent girls experiencing sexual pleasure. Fortunately, the inner areas of the clitoris are less likely to be damaged by clitoridectomy, leaving some women able to experience an orgasm, anyway.

Physical conditions that may affect orgasm are more likely to be found in women who used to be able to orgasm and now find it difficult to do so. See chapter 5 for more information on these conditions.

## RATING

HOW much influence do you think **physical conditions** have had on your sexual feelings? (Without a medical check, you can only guess at this.)

| Influence in the past: | Influence now: |
| --- | --- |
| ❐ A great deal | ❐ A great deal |
| ❐ Quite a lot | ❐ Quite a lot |
| ❐ Some | ❐ Some |
| ❐ A little | ❐ A little |
| ❐ None | ❐ None |

## conclusions

I'M TOLD BY many women who never or rarely feel orgasm that they've been given all sorts of tests for medical and hormonal conditions in the search to find the cause of their difficulties.

But, as you can see, most of the reasons for your situation involve psychological and lifestyle issues. Your difficulty is more likely to have been learned, either when you were a child or as you began to explore your sexuality. What you learned can be stated very simply:

**You learned how to stop your feelings of sexual pleasure from becoming stronger.**

And, as you now know, this will stop you from having an orgasm.

☙

HOPEFULLY, THIS CHAPTER has helped you to have a better understanding of yourself. Try not to be discouraged as a result of what you've learned here.

Being able to pinpoint the cause of your orgasm difficulties is a very important step. As I've said before, *self-understanding and self-awareness are the first steps to change.* You can't sort out any kind of personal difficulty without these two ingredients.

With a better understanding of what causes your orgasm difficulties, you now have somewhere to start in your quest to become more sexually aroused. We'll move on to programs for changing your situation later in this book.

## BUT WAIT!

Before you flip over the pages, I suggest you read through the next two chapters which look at causes of other types of orgasm difficulties. You never know which piece of information will help in understanding your own situation. Be open to learning all you can about yourself.

**A final point:** If after reading this chapter, you feel unsure as to which of the causes seems to fit your situation, it might be useful to see a psychologist or professional counselor specializing in sexuality. He or she can go through the points with you and help to sort out what seems to have influenced your difficulties with sexual arousal.

# what changed?
## women who used to have orgasms (and now don't)

CAN YOU THINK back to a time when you could regularly orgasm (yet don't feel anything now)? Do you remember when having an orgasm happened naturally (but now it seems hard work to reach high levels of arousal)? Were your orgasms once strong and enjoyable (but now are so weak that you barely notice them)?

If you answered yes to any of these questions, you're probably wondering why you don't climax the way you used to. In this chapter I would like to help you find the answer to your question.

So let's talk about *when* your sexual feelings changed and *what* changed.

---

*Well, I just woke up the other day and thought,
hey, I've got a problem with orgasms. I can now see
that it's been like this for a while. I haven't any idea
what happened, but I feel a bit embarrassed with
the whole thing.*

---

Don't be. It's often hard to see what's happening in our lives. Besides, with so many other things needing our attention, it's no wonder that sexual reactions can be easily ignored. If your difficulty with sexual arousal happened suddenly, you might have noticed the change. But, for many women, it's a *gradual* change, so it's easy to miss what's going on until much later.

Now that you've realized your orgasms are missing or difficult to feel, you can begin to find out why this is happening. To help you get started, I've given you a short quiz about the changes in your life. Take some time to think back; it doesn't matter how far you go. Write your answers here or in your notebook.

## a quiz about change

1. When did you stop having orgasms?

_____

2. Was the change sudden or gradual?

_____

3. Where were you in your life when the changes began:

_____

Where were you living?

_____

Who was with you at this time?

_____

What job were you in?

_____

What events were occurring?

_____

There are so many things that shift and change in our lives. Relationships come and go, children leave home, people die, we change jobs (or lose them), move house or town *or* country, grow up, grow old, experience a traumatic event, travel, and so on. The list could go on forever. However, it's not actual events that prevent sexual arousal from building. Rather, it's your *emotional and mental reactions* to those events and changes.

In the rest of this chapter, I've described how this can happen.

# causes of orgasm difficulties:
## women who used to be able to orgasm

**Cause #13:** Life became full of stress and upset
**Cause #14:** Life became boring
**Cause #15:** Less time taken to become aroused
**Cause #16:** Sex became painful
**Cause #17:** Changes to health

# CAUSE #13: |
## life became full of stress and upset

WHEN STRESSFUL EVENTS happen in our lives, we usually feel strong emotion, such as worry, anxiety, and grief. Actually, any strong emotion can affect sexual arousal. Stress, anxiety, rage, and worry, not to mention panic, nervousness, and depression, are good examples of feelings that will affect sexual arousal. So, too, are grief and hurt.

These emotions *compete* with and *replace* sexual arousal. How can this happen? Quite easily, I'm afraid. If you feel anxiety, grief or any of the emotions I've just mentioned, your focus will be on whatever is troubling you. You'll think about something that happened recently, or in the distant past. Or you'll have your mind on what's going to happen in the future. Your muscles will then probably tighten in reaction to your thoughts and emotions, leaving you tense and uncomfortable. Do you feel sexy with all this going on? I doubt it!

For most of us, it's just impossible to feel strong emotions like this *and* still feel sexy. Try thinking of emotional stress and sexual arousal as *opposites*, and you'll see what I mean. They simply cancel each other out. Remember what I said earlier: in order to feel sexual arousal (especially *high* sexual arousal), we need to be relaxed and ready to enjoy ourselves. This is hard to do if you're knotted up with worry or sadness.

**In other words, dear reader, some emotions are very effective *passion killers*.**

Take a moment to see if you can identify any passion-killers in your life at present. Place a cross next to those you're experiencing now.

## PASSION-KILLER EMOTIONS
- ❏ Stress
- ❏ Anxiety
- ❏ Worry
- ❏ Feeling down
- ❏ Panic
- ❏ Concern
- ❏ Resentment
- ❏ Disappointment
- ❏ Frustration
- ❏ Grief
- ❏ Emotional hurt
- ❏ Fear
- ❏ Sadness
- ❏ Shame
- ❏ Other

Now, think over the life events or changes that have occurred in recent days, weeks, months or even years that seem to be creating these emotions. Make a list of these events or changes.

## changes occurring in my life
### that make me feel stressed and upset

1. _____

2. _____

3. _____

4. _____

Next, see if you can work out which of these events took place around the time you began to have difficulties with orgasm. It doesn't have to be on an exact day.

Here are some examples of life events and changes that I've seen affecting women:

- a promotion at work that meant extra responsibilities and longer hours
- trouble with a neighbor that threatened to end up in court
- a child becoming ill and needing hospitalization
- a pregnancy termination
- separating from a partner
- the sudden death of a parent or family member
- sexual harassment or abuse
- relationship problems
- struggling to pay the bills
- having a baby
- a partner retiring
- moving to another country
- becoming ill
- losing friends

There are so many things that can upset our routine or sense of peace, put extra pressure on us and then leave us with strong passion-killer emotions.

Yes, but everyone has something like this happen
to them. Do they ALL have difficulties with orgasm?

Good point. And the answer is no. These things don't automatically have to affect our sex life.

Somehow, this doesn't make me feel so great!

No, I suppose it doesn't. The truth is that some people, like you,
are more affected than others. That doesn't mean that you're less of
a person. But it may mean that your way of coping with stress or
emotions might need rethinking so that it won't stop you from building sexual arousal.

Keep in mind, however, there isn't a woman alive who hasn't, at
some time, had trouble getting aroused when tired, stressed, or sad.
It's a perfectly natural reaction.

Ongoing orgasm difficulties seem to occur when the stress or
upset continues over a period of time. Once again, however, some
people seem to ride out the tough times better than others. These
women usually deal with emotions by talking out their problems
with others.

They probably have a good cry (or a yell) when things get a bit
too much. And they'll be prepared to go to friends or partners for a
hug and a bit of support. Women who cope in this way are much less
likely to have their sexual feelings seriously affected by what's happening in their lives.

That's all very well, but I'm not one to talk about my
feelings. In fact, I don't have a partner to share with at the
moment. And I get embarrassed even thinking about
asking for a hug. Don't you think that if my friends were
caring enough, they'd make the time to call without my
asking? Anyway, I was brought up to be independent and
solve everything myself, rather than burden others.

Whew! You don't make it easy for yourself, do you? All I can tell you is that bottling things up inside may stop you from feeling vulnerable, but it'll also create a huge buildup of all the stress and upset feelings. Something like an emotional log jam. And then your feelings will just get stronger and stronger until you feel ready to burst.

It takes a lot of energy to try and control what's going on inside while pretending to others you're doing fine. One thing's for sure, it's not a coping style that'll make you relaxed and ready to let your sexual feelings go.

You may not have realized it, but pushing down feelings such as anxiety and grief can lead to all feelings being squashed down—*including sexual ones.* It's hard to choose some feelings to be hidden away and some to be kept out in the open.

I picture it like this:

> MESSAGE FROM CONTROL TO BASE: *Send up the Happy and Sexy feelings. I repeat, ONLY the Happy and Sexy ones. No, no Anger, stay down there. You, too, Worry. Didn't you hear? I only want Happy and Sexy feelings.*

> REPLY FROM BASE TO CONTROL: *Sorry, no can do. There's too much Stress and Upset down here to let the Happy and Sexy feelings through. It's a real log jam, I can tell you.*

Sound familiar?

In reality, women who bottle up feelings can sometimes get a *little* turned on (in other words, a small amount of "Happy" and "Sexy" feelings can occasionally squeeze through the log jam for a short period). But as for really letting go and moving up the arousal hill towards orgasm, forget it. It doesn't happen.

And another thing. You may be stopping your sexual pleasure from building to orgasm in order to keep other emotions from getting through. Letting down barriers to express *one* emotion can allow *others* to pour out (see my earlier discussion of this in chapter 4, Cause #3).

A good example of this is the way women sometimes cry as they have an orgasm. Remember, at the moment of orgasm, we let go of emotional control for a few moments. So, any tears stored up from an upsetting event can pop out alongside the orgasm. You may have sensed that this can happen, leading to your keeping your sexual pleasure under control.

I should add that having a good cry with orgasm can leave you feeling quite relaxed and peaceful. And it's rather nice if you can snuffle into the shoulder of a partner who wants to comfort you (but some women hate being this vulnerable).

**Just one final point:** Whenever we push down or *depress* our feelings over a period of time, we run the risk of ending up feeling flat and lifeless (or depressed). If this happens, then sexual arousal is even more difficult to build to orgasm levels.

Depression usually makes us feel too miserable to get more than a little turned on. It also leaves us lacking in energy (to keep climbing the arousal hill). And more importantly, because depression takes away our motivation, we don't really care whether we have an orgasm or not.

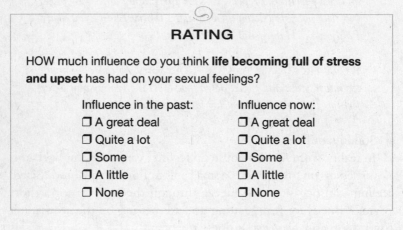

### RATING

HOW much influence do you think **life becoming full of stress and upset** has had on your sexual feelings?

| Influence in the past: | Influence now: |
|---|---|
| ❏ A great deal | ❏ A great deal |
| ❏ Quite a lot | ❏ Quite a lot |
| ❏ Some | ❏ Some |
| ❏ A little | ❏ A little |
| ❏ None | ❏ None |

## CAUSE #14:
### life became boring

LET ME NOW turn to something a little different. I've met many women who suddenly realized that their lives had become very dull and boring. Even sex had become boring.

**If you think boredom won't affect your sexual arousal, think again.**

There are two ways in which boredom plays a part in sexual enjoyment. Firstly, if you allow yourself to slip into a boring lifestyle, or *you* become a dull and predictable person, then your sex life will probably become boring, too. The dullness will simply spread to everything you do.

It's not easy admitting you've become boring. Or that your life holds no excitement. Yet, it may be the first step to understanding your orgasm difficulties.

Why don't you try the Boredom Quiz I've set out below?

## boredom quiz

1. Do you ever wonder what happened to the excitement in your life?

   Yes ☐    No ☐

2. Do you lack hobbies, activities, or events that you really look forward to?

   Yes ☐    No ☐

3. How long ago did you get a buzz out of hobbies, activities or events:

   ☐ two years    ☐ ten years    ☐ you hate to think

4. When did you last do something quite spontaneous?

   ☐ last 6 months    ☐ 1 to 2 years ago    ☐ can't remember

   Is it likely to happen again in the near future?    Yes ☐    No ☐

5. Are you so caught up in the day-to-day grind that you've forgotten how to have fun?

   Yes ☐    No ☐

6. Has everything in your life become routine?

   Yes ☐    No ☐

7. Do you catch yourself dreaming about exciting people and events?

   Yes ☐    No ☐

If the answer was yes to two or more of these questions, then I think you know the problem. In this case, your orgasm difficulties are only a symptom of the bigger issue: the lack of pep in your life.

The second way in which boredom stops us from having orgasms is quite simple, really. If you no longer bring fun and new ideas into your lovemaking, it becomes predictable and—you guessed it—boring. To be exciting, or at least interesting, sex needs to be playful, spontaneous, and fun.

Can you describe exactly what's going to happen during sex? If so, then sex has definitely become too routine and predictable. When this happens, our sexual triggers stop working, and we struggle to get turned on. It's hard to feel sexually interested when you know what's going to happen from the moment you start having sex.

Absolutely! It's like following a recipe: the ingredients are the same, and so is the cooking process. Touch here, touch there. More of the same. Climax. How exciting is that?

My point, exactly.

Now, think about when sex first began to be predictable. Can you remember when this happened? The trouble is, we often don't realize we're getting into a rut *until we're in it*.

For many women it starts something like this: You're tired. Too tired for sex. Or you're busy and don't have enough time for sex. But you're feeling sexy (or maybe your partner is), so the easiest thing to do is to keep it simple—a bit of touching, build the arousal, have an orgasm, collapse onto the pillow, then off to sleep. Do that often enough and you'll forget that "once upon a time" sex used to be passionate, sensual and varied.

The same thing can happen with masturbation if you do it using the same fantasy and the same method. Very quickly it becomes a habit, rather than an enjoyable activity.

The problem with doing things in a predictable and familiar way is that sexual feelings become numbed. There's nothing happening to stimulate your sexual triggers. You can probably get a little aroused when your clitoris is touched, but with none of your other senses getting involved, this won't be enough to orgasm.

Many women find the thought of trying something different rather scary. You may be shy or unadventurous. You may not know what to do to bring some excitement into your sexual contacts. The thought of suggesting new sexual ways to a partner may fill you with anxiety or guilt. Perhaps you once tried to bring up the topic without success and now feel too embarrassed to try again.

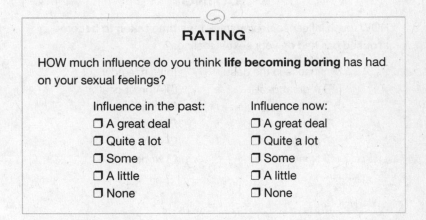

## RATING

HOW much influence do you think **life becoming boring** has had on your sexual feelings?

| Influence in the past: | Influence now: |
| --- | --- |
| ❑ A great deal | ❑ A great deal |
| ❑ Quite a lot | ❑ Quite a lot |
| ❑ Some | ❑ Some |
| ❑ A little | ❑ A little |
| ❑ None | ❑ None |

# CAUSE #15:
## less time taken to become aroused

THIS IS VERY similar to Cause #6. One of the most common changes in women's lives is that they become *too* busy. And when this happens, sex is given little importance. Less time is spent thinking about sex and, more importantly, *being* sexual.

Instead of an enjoyable, relaxing moment, sex becomes rushed. It may be squeezed in at the end of the day or between other things that need to be done. The aim is to do it in the time available. This means there's little chance you'll be able to relax and slowly wind down from a busy day. You'll still be acting and thinking like a "mother," "career woman," "wife," or "employee," instead of "lover," "partner" or "sexual woman."

Remember the stages of arousal I described in chapter 3? Getting turned on takes time. Time for you to relax. And time for you to get in a sexual mood. Unless you're in a new sexual situation (which can trigger sexual pleasure more quickly), quick sex may leave you feeling nothing but frustration.

You'd be surprised how many women start having orgasms again when they make a point of extending their sexual time by even twenty minutes of gentle caressing, massaging or talking (but more on this later).

---

### RATING

HOW much influence do you think **less time taken to become aroused** has had on your sexual feelings?

| Influence in the past: | Influence now: |
|---|---|
| ❐ A great deal | ❐ A great deal |
| ❐ Quite a lot | ❐ Quite a lot |
| ❐ Some | ❐ Some |
| ❐ A little | ❐ A little |
| ❐ None | ❐ None |

---

## CAUSE #16: |
### sex became painful

IT'S NOT OFTEN that the effects of pain are discussed in relation to sexual arousal. Yet, when pain occurs during sex, it can have an enormous effect. We quickly go from enjoying sexual feelings and orgasms to recoiling from anything that hints of sex.

Pain can affect your willingness to be touched, the types of sexual activities you enjoy, the level of sexual arousal you can tolerate, your ability to relax and focus on sexual pleasure, and so on. In other words, pain can make it difficult to want or to enjoy sexual feelings.

Women feel pain in the sexual situation for several reasons. Some examples are:

- any medical condition (such as an infection) that makes the vulva, clitoris, vagina, or nipples sore to touch. Thrush is a common example. Allergies to soap, creams or chemicals can also create soreness. Conditions causing nerve damage or affecting skin sensitivity, such as vulvodynia or vulvar vestibulitis, can also lead to pain.

- any condition that causes joint stiffness and makes movement painful. Women with arthritis are well aware of this problem.
- any condition that makes it hard to relax the entrance of the vagina. Scar tissue from surgery after giving birth is a good example. Muscle tension caused by fear and anxiety is another.
- an intact hymen. Not common, but occasionally found in young women. Some women have a thick hymen that does not break during vaginal or other forms of penetration.
- any rough touching of the vulva, clitoris or vagina that tears or inflames the skin. A partner's rough skin (for example, on the hands) can make this happen .
- vaginal dryness caused by menopause. If lubrication isn't used, any movement against the walls of the vagina from penis, vibrator, dildo or even tampon may tear the skin.
- thinning of the skin on the vulva, clitoris or vagina (caused by menopause and some medical conditions) that can lead to pain, if the skin is not touched gently and lubrication used.
- soreness from too much sexual activity.
- soreness or pain caused by sexual activity that is beyond the body's capabilities. This may be due to a lack of fitness, a difference in the body size of partners, a difference in genital size (for example, a women with a short vagina having sexual intercourse with a man with an unusually long penis or a penis that is bent).
- the presence of injury or disease that creates ill health in areas of the body used during sexual arousal and sexual activity. For example, chronic pelvic infection; diseases of the bladder, uterus, and ovaries; multiple sclerosis.
- any disability or injury producing general chronic pain during sexual activity, which cannot easily be relieved by painkillers.

- pelvic congestion. Sexual arousal without orgasm can lead to pelvic pain or to the clitoris becoming extremely sensitive.
- headaches at orgasm.

Pain can have two important effects on our enjoyment of sex. First, it's distracting. Our attention shifts from sexual pleasure to coping with the pain.

---

I know what you mean. I just can't concentrate on
enjoying sex when I'm hurting. It really upsets me—
the pain always seems to be stronger than any
sexual feelings I get.

---

Yes, pain is hard to ignore. It makes it difficult to relax and let your sexual arousal build to the levels needed for you to orgasm.

Pain has another effect on our sexual arousal. It leads to a *fear of pain*. Just think for a moment about the first time you felt pain during sex. It caught you by surprise, didn't it? Aah, but not the next time. You were ready for it. Waiting, tensed up in case it happened again. Who wouldn't be? Few of us like pain, so it's natural to stiffen up if you think it might happen again.

However, as you now know, being anxious and tense can bring sexual arousal to a grinding halt. It's hard to concentrate on enjoying sexual pleasure if all you can think of is whether sex is going to hurt!

**So, the fear of pain becomes the problem.**

The truth is, fear is probably responsible for more pain experienced during sex than actual infections or other physical conditions. It will make you tense and unable to relax your body. You'll be sensitive, but it's likely to be an uncomfortable sensitivity, not the enjoyable type you feel when sexually aroused. And because the entrance to your vagina is surrounded by muscle, it too will become tight. Any attempt at vaginal penetration will then result in pain.

To make matters worse, when you're tense and anxious, there's a good chance you won't lubricate, or become wet, in the vagina. In that way, a fear of pain will also lead to dryness, and dryness can lead to actual pain. We usually need some wetness to help a finger, penis, body, or other object slide easily over our skin. With dryness the skin may tear or be rubbed raw, causing soreness and pain.

❧

GENITAL DRYNESS IS a common cause of pain in young women. If you've only just begun your sexual experiences, you may find that having your vagina entered is quite painful. Touching of your vulva and clitoris may also hurt.

There may be several reasons for this. Perhaps you're feeling anxious about the whole sexual situation. Perhaps you lack confidence about what to do. Perhaps you had intercourse (had a penis in your vagina) when you were just starting up the arousal hill and weren't emotionally and physically ready.

Whatever the cause, if you're tense and can't relax, then it's unlikely you'll be able to get aroused enough to stay wet. This is likely to lead to pain, unless saliva or artificial lubrication is used (the latter can be obtained from pharmacies, drug stores and supermarkets).

❧

I WOULD NOW like to make a switch and talk to older women who have reached menopause. The situation here is a little different. You may be ready, willing and able when it comes to sex, but are unable to lubricate easily because of the low levels of hormones (estrogen and androgens) in your body.

If you're in this situation and try to have sex without using something to moisten your vulva, clitoris, and vagina (such as massage oil or a lubricant), it's likely to irritate the skin and make it sore.

Another very common cause of the pain older women sometimes feel during sexual activity is a lower level of fitness. As we lose muscle tone in our stomach, legs, and back (in fact, throughout our whole body), we find ourselves less able to do the things we used to do.

The trouble is, your head may think you can do it, whereas your body can't keep up. So, if you're trying to make love as you did when you were in your twenties or thirties, watch out. Pulled muscles and torn ligaments can be awfully embarrassing to explain.

*Well, you see doctor, it was like this. I was . . . ah . . . in bed and . . . ah . . . I . . . moved into this . . . ah . . . interesting position . . . and oh, it hurt . . .*

Not a situation many of us would like to see ourselves in!

∾

THERE'S JUST ONE more piece of information about pain and sex you should know. It seems that our bodies have excellent "memories" when it comes to pain. Even when the condition that originally caused it has long gone, *our body remembers.* Boy, does it remember! Without even realizing it, you'll begin to tense up in readiness for the pain. Your body (or at least your brain) remembers how the pain used to feel. It's a kind of safety mechanism your mind has adopted to protect you from further pain.

Fear of pain can be something you're fully aware of, or it can be so deep down in your unconscious, you don't know it's there.

---

## RATING

HOW much influence do you think **sex becoming painful** has had on your sexual feelings

| Influence in the past: | Influence now: |
|---|---|
| ❐ A great deal | ❐ A great deal |
| ❐ Quite a lot | ❐ Quite a lot |
| ❐ Some | ❐ Some |
| ❐ A little | ❐ A little |
| ❐ None | ❐ None |

---

# CAUSE #17:
## changes to health

LOSS OF HEALTH can play a part in whether we orgasm or not. One study found that women in poor health were nearly *twice* as likely to have orgasm difficulties as women in excellent health (36.7% compared to 20.2%).[10]

Some **medical diseases and physical conditions** can make it difficult for women to have an orgasm, or can make their orgasm less pleasurable. This can happen when the disease or condition:

- stops or reduces the blood flow to the genitals
- damages the nerves to the genital and nipple area
- reduces the tone and fitness of muscles involved in sexual arousal and orgasm
- lowers the levels of hormones that affect sensitivity, arousal and lubrication
- makes it difficult to stay in a sexual situation because of pain, fatigue, spasms, etc.
- changes genital skin sensitivity

This means that the normal physical reactions that take place during arousal and lead to orgasm don't occur. For example, your clitoris may become less sensitive and even feel numb. You may be unable to get wet. Your orgasm may be weaker and take longer to reach.

Now, let me be clear. These conditions MAY cause orgasm difficulties. I did not say they WILL cause orgasm difficulties. It all depends on how severe the disease or condition is. Women with mild forms may not experience sexual difficulties at all.

Let me give you some examples of these diseases and conditions:

- diabetes mellitus, which may cause damage to the nerves or blood supply of the clitoris
- neurological conditions (such as multiple sclerosis and polio) that damage the spinal cord and other nerves, and may cause loss of sensitivity in the vulva, clitoris and pelvic areas
- neurological conditions caused by severe malnutrition and vitamin deficiencies
- injury to the spinal cord and other nerves linked to feeling orgasm (e.g., paraplegia, quadriplegia)
- spinal degeneration, which injures the nerves controlling orgasm

- injury to the pelvic and spinal area caused by surgery (e.g., for rectal, cervical or bladder cancers, hysterectomy), childbirth, falls (e.g., off a bicycle or horse), and aging
- thyroid deficiencies and other endocrine disorders (e.g., Addison's disease)
- liver disease (e.g., hepatitis), and kidney disease
- androgen (e.g., testosterone, DHEA) deficiencies that may reduce clitoral sensitivity and possibly an interest in sex
- vulval conditions (e.g. cancer of the vulva or clitoris, Lichen Sclerosus, vulvodynia
- brain tumors and head injury, epilepsy
- adhesions of the clitoris hood
- nerve damage as a result of alcoholism
- weakness of the pelvic muscles (often due to childbirth or aging)
- high cholesterol, high blood pressure, and heart disease, which damage blood vessels and restrict blood flow
- heavy smoking that damages blood flow
- nerve and blood vessel damage caused by excessive bicycle or horse riding
- menopause, leading to low levels of estrogen and androgens
- pregnancy, from about six months on.
- heavy use of some drugs (e.g., heroin), which reduce lubrication and clitoral sensitivity

Now, I realize that *at this very moment* some of you will be rushing to the phone to make an appointment with your doctor. Especially those of you who tend to assume there's a physical or medical cause for *all* your ailments (you know who you are).

JUST HOLD IT! Now, please read the next sentence.

**It's not very common for women's orgasm difficulties to be related to medical problems.**

Your difficulties are far more likely to have a psychological or social cause than a physical one.

If you've already been diagnosed with a medical condition and your doctor hasn't discussed the kinds of sexual difficulties it may cause, you should check it out. Don't be put off by a bland or superficial answer, either. If your doctor doesn't seem to know (or is embarrassed by your question), try to find someone who specializes in sexual medicine.

However, some medical conditions rarely get diagnosed until a woman complains of loss of sexual feelings or loss of the ability to get aroused. An example of this is damage to the nerves connected to the clitoris, which occurs during surgery to the pelvic or genital area.

**And another thing:** changes to our physical health often bring psychological reactions. You may experience a great sense of loss at feeling less sexual. You may find it hard to see yourself as a sexual person or a woman any more. Changes to your body may be hard to accept. Your partner may have difficulty accepting the changes to your health. And so on.

So far I've talked about *physical* changes to your health. Changes to your **mental health** can also make it difficult to orgasm or make the orgasm less enjoyable. Mental conditions can:

- make it difficult to concentrate during sexual activity, resulting in us cutting off arousal
- stop us from having strong feelings of pleasure and enjoyment
- stop us being relaxed enough to allow arousal to build.

Once again, please note, I said changes to mental health *can* make it difficult to orgasm—not *will* make it difficult to orgasm. In fact, some women with mental health changes aren't affected in this way. Examples of the types of mental health conditions that *may* stop you from enjoying orgasms are:

- depression
- anxiety, including panic attacks, agoraphobia, and obsessive-compulsive behavior
- posttraumatic stress
- hypermania and manic depression (bipolar disorder)

- psychosis
- dissociative conditions.

---

> Well, I used to be able to orgasm easily, but now I
> have a panic attack as soon as I get turned on. I
> feel my heart going faster and then I can't
> concentrate or relax.

---

Many women with high levels of anxiety become scared when their heart begins to race. It's thinking negative thoughts that usually makes this happen, but highly anxious people often think it's a sign of a heart attack. They then become *more* anxious, which can lead to a panic attack.

◡

SOMETIMES IT'S NOT so much a physical or mental condition that stops us from having an orgasm, but the **medications** we take for them.

Some medications and drugs, such as antidepressants, can make it difficult for women to reach orgasm.[11]

Women on antidepressants often feel they're stuck on a plateau that is almost at the top of their arousal hill, and no matter how much they try, they can't go any further. Their orgasm seems to be just beyond reach, or else takes forever to come.

---

> I know exactly what you're talking about.
> And, let me tell you, there is only one word
> for this—frustrating.

---

Actually, *frustrating* is a word I've heard many women use in this situation. What's even more frustrating is that women are often given these kinds of medications without a *single* word from the doctor about the possible effects on their sexual arousal. They become aroused but find it impossible to reach a climax (or can do so only after a *long* time of constant touching). Not realizing it's the medication, they keep trying and trying, and end up feeling confused (and exhausted). Naturally, they begin to believe there's something wrong with themselves or their partner. It's a great sense of relief once they know it's not their "fault."

I should add, however, that some antidepressants (especially those called SSRIs) seem to affect sexual arousal whereas others don't. Furthermore, higher doses of some antidepressants have an effect, but lower doses don't. Interestingly, I've spoken with women using the same antidepressant and found that, while some were affected sexually, others were not.

There is another way that depression can make it difficult for women to orgasm. It can leave you feeling tired, lacking in energy and unmotivated. It's hard to stay interested and involved with sex when you feel like this. Not surprisingly, your level of arousal will probably be low, and without high levels of sexual arousal, orgasm just won't happen.

There are many medications and drugs that may affect a woman's sexual arousal. Check out the list below:

- antidepressants—such as SSRIs
- sedatives, such as barbituates, temazepam
- some antianxiety drugs/tranquilizers, such as diazepam
- narcotics, such as codeine and morphine
- opiates, such as heroin
- stimulants, such as cocaine and amphetamines
- some antihypertensive drugs, for high blood pressure
- some medications for psychosis
- beta adrenergic blockers
- some anticancer drugs
- alcohol

The effects of these drugs and medications can be different in different women. You could have no difficulty with orgasm *or* be unable to orgasm at all *or* have less intense or less frequent orgasms, *or* even have spontaneous orgasms when you're least expecting them.

Once again, if you're not sure whether your sexual arousal is being affected by drugs or medications, check with your doctor. Keep in mind, however, that the sexual side effects are better known for some drugs/medications than others. Do *not* suddenly stop taking any medications. You may end up with a reaction that's much worse than loss of orgasm!

@

THERE IS ONE more thing you need to know. Our mental and physical *reactions* to illness can also put a dampener on our willingness to become aroused. Some women, for example, report feeling less aroused after a heart attack, but this is more likely to be due to *concern* about their health rather than actual physical damage. Although they fear a rise in blood pressure at orgasm, the truth is that blood pressure is usually higher during moderate *non*sexual activity.

A painful or restricting medical condition such as arthritis can also make it difficult to reach high levels of arousal because the difficulty in moving during sexual activity breaks the sexual mood.

Some women find it hard to adjust to the changes in their health. They feel angry, self-conscious about their bodies, despairing, sad, awkward, cheated, frustrated, ugly, and so on. These kinds of emotions, and the negative thoughts behind them, can quite overpower the sexual feelings. So, if you're in the middle of making love and start thinking about your illness, don't be surprised if shortly afterwards you begin to lose concentration and find your sexual arousal disappearing.

Finally, difficulties may arise if your partner suggests sex when you're not feeling well enough to enjoy it. If you go along with the suggestion, without saying honestly how you're feeling, the likely result will be resentment on your part or a distraction from your sexual feelings caused by the pain or discomfort.

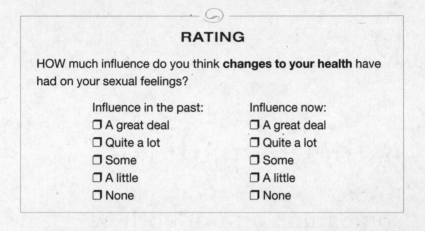

**RATING**

HOW much influence do you think **changes to your health** have had on your sexual feelings?

Influence in the past:
- ❏ A great deal
- ❏ Quite a lot
- ❏ Some
- ❏ A little
- ❏ None

Influence now:
- ❏ A great deal
- ❏ Quite a lot
- ❏ Some
- ❏ A little
- ❏ None

## conclusions |

LIFE EVENTS AND personal changes play a big part in the way we feel about ourselves and our partners. If things become too much, we soon react. We shut down our emotions, withdraw into ourselves, and tense up physically.

As you now know, anything which causes us to shut down our emotions can also shut down our sexual arousal and stop us from having an orgasm.

So, if you're no longer able to orgasm, look on it as a SIGN that you need to stop and take notice. Something is happening in your life, and it shouldn't be ignored.

# 6

## is there a pattern?
### women who can orgasm at some times and not others

WHAT DOES IT feel like to be able to orgasm at some times and not at others? For some women it can be confusing, for others frustrating (that word pops up again and again, doesn't it?). Some see it as a problem that needs to be fixed, while others don't care whether or not they orgasm on every occasion.

---

Well, I'm not sure if I have a problem or not. I know I can't expect to always climax, but it seems impossible for me to predict what's going to happen. Sometimes I can get really turned on and orgasm, sometimes I can't. Is that normal?

---

Mmm . . . I get very jittery when someone starts to talk about what's normal in women's orgasms. There are so many different ways in which women feel sexual and have orgasms that it's just impossible to say something is *normal* or not.

However, I will say that in one investigation, only about a quarter of the women studied (27.1%) said that in the previous twelve months they had *always* had an orgasm during sexual activity. Of the remainder, nearly a quarter (21.6%) said they could orgasm at *some* times, but not at others.[12] These findings seem to apply whether the sexual activity is with a partner or not.[13] We certainly don't get the impression that being able to orgasm at some times and not others is unusual, do we? Quite the opposite! It seems to be the experience of one in six women.

However, it doesn't really matter how many other women have orgasm difficulties on some occasions. What matters is *you* and how you feel about your situation. Some women are quite happy expressing themselves sexually without having an orgasm. In fact, of the women mentioned earlier who sometimes had orgasms in the previous twelve months, *half* (50.9%) described themselves as extremely or very happy.[14]

So, let's start with what *you* think. If you feel that your lack of orgasms is a difficulty, then it *is*—for *you* (and if you're quite happy with the way you express your sexual feelings, you don't need this book).

I hope it's now clear that in this chapter I'm not going to worry about how often you *should* orgasm. Instead, I want to get you thinking about your **orgasm patterns**. There's often a pattern to when women can and can't become completely aroused. Finding this pattern is the first step in understanding your difficulties with orgasm.

The second step is identifying the causes of your pattern. Read on, and let's see what you can discover about yourself.

## you could be like everyone else |

BEFORE LOOKING FOR orgasm patterns, I want to repeat my message in chapter 1 that *any* woman can have difficulty becoming aroused enough to orgasm. This is a very, very common occurrence.

Have you ever been in a situation that is usually sexually arousing for you, only to realize you were unable to get turned on enough to reach orgasm?

Perhaps you were tired to begin with . . .
*(and didn't think to say no),*

or unwell . . .
*(and didn't think to say no),*

Maybe you had something on your mind . . .
*(and didn't think to say no),*

or got distracted during sex by the baby crying or the phone ringing . . .
*(and didn't think to stop and have a cup of tea instead).*

We turn off during sex for a million reasons (well, maybe not a million exactly, but more than I can list here, that's for sure). Every woman has probably experienced one of them at some time.

---

Well, I can tell you, distraction is a REAL problem for me. The slightest little noise and my sexual feelings disappear out the window. I'm just too sensitive, I guess.

---

No, you're not *too* sensitive—just tuned into your surroundings, as are a lot of other women. The truth is, most women are sensitive to what's going on around them during sex. As a result, they're easily put off. Men don't seem to have this problem to the same degree. I'm not sure if they're the luckier ones, or we are.

Anyway, there's nothing to get worried about unless it happens more often than you'd like or if you can't come right out and say, *I don't feel like sex/orgasms today.*

There's nothing wrong with being unable to get aroused or orgasm. It *is* a problem, though, if you can't be assertive enough to say when you're not in the mood.

*To put it in a nutshell,* if you can look back and see that,

• your difficulty with orgasm seems to occur quite often

- there seems to be a pattern to the occasions when you can and can't orgasm
- and—I repeat, *and*—this pattern presents problems for you,

then you may find the rest of this chapter useful.

# patterns of not being able to orgasm |

I'VE FOUND THAT most patterns for women who don't always orgasm can actually be summarised under three headings:

**1. Being able to orgasm in some situations, but not others**
*Some examples:*
- A woman who could only orgasm in the kitchen
- A woman who could never orgasm the first time she had sex with someone
- A woman who could only orgasm if lovemaking occurred at night
- A woman who could only orgasm when she and her parents were living in different cities

**2. Being able to orgasm during some sexual activities, but not others**
*Some examples:*
- A woman who could never orgasm during intercourse
- A woman who could never orgasm during sex with a partner, but could do so quite easily on her own
- A woman who could only orgasm with someone who was very forceful

**3. Being able to orgasm with some people, or some kinds of people, but not others**
*Some examples:*
- A woman who could orgasm with a lover, but never her long-term partner

- A woman who could orgasm with a female, but never a male partner
- A woman who could only orgasm with someone who was already in a relationship (with someone else)
- A woman who could only orgasm with a partner whom she saw as especially manly or macho

What these examples tell us is that some *situations,* some *sexual activities,* and some *types of people* trigger our sexual feelings, while others cause us to switch off sexually. This can happen to any of us and shouldn't necessarily be seen as a problem. Here are some examples of patterns that are not a problem:

- A young woman of twenty who knows that she isn't sexually attracted to someone thirty years older *(and doesn't want to change this)*
- A woman who is aware she isn't really turned on by a man's body *(and doesn't want to change this)*
- A woman who finds black skin very sexy *(and doesn't want to change this)*

These people see their turn-on/turn-off pattern as acceptable. They have no wish to change it and are content to get aroused or to orgasm only at those times when their sexual feelings are triggered.

However, if our pattern of sexual arousal makes us uncomfortable or makes our life difficult, we may not be so content. For example, if you enjoy orgasms when participating in oral sex, but feel pressured by a partner to have them during intercourse, you may feel angry because he doesn't care about your needs.

If you're in a relationship with a man, and become strongly attracted to another woman, you may be left trying to explain why you're having trouble getting turned on with him now. If you're happy to masturbate to orgasm, but don't care if you orgasm with your partner, he or she may demand an explanation.

The point is, *someone* will probably be upset in these kinds of situations. Perhaps it will be your partner who's wondering why your sexual arousal isn't the same on every occasion. Perhaps it will be you who's concerned about the times you can't reach high levels of arousal.

So, if being able to orgasm at some times and not others seems a problem for you, then read on and see if you can understand a little more of why you are the way you are.

## your turn-on and turn-off patterns |

LET'S BEGIN BY trying to understand something about your arousal patterns. Do you know what your turn-on/turn-off pattern is? If you haven't given much thought to it before, try the exercise below. See if you can identify which situations, activities and types of people turn you on and off sexually. (By the way, everyone should try this exercise, even if they don't have this particular orgasm difficulty; it can be a real eye-opener.)

---

## identifying your turn-on and turn-off patterns
### Instructions:

Under the heading, **Turn On**, make a list of situations, activities and types of people that allow you to become sexually aroused. Under the heading, **Turn Off**, make a list of situations, activities and types of people that keep you from becoming sexually aroused.

|  | Turn On | Turn Off |
|---|---|---|
| Sexual situations (Where/When you have sex) |  |  |
| Sexual activities (What you do sexually) |  |  |
| Types of people (Who you have sex with) |  |  |

Now sit for a moment and look at what you've written. Many women have never taken the time to think about what gets them sexually excited or otherwise.

It really is important to find out what makes you tick sexually. We all have one set of conditions that trigger feelings of sexual pleasure and another set that will switch off these feelings. Some women don't know enough about their sexual arousal patterns to recognize which set is which. If they get into a sexual situation that doesn't arouse them, it's assumed they're doing something wrong. They mistakenly blame their lack of personality, skills, or attractiveness, when it may be that the atmosphere is wrong, their partner unattractive, or the sexual activities unexciting.

For example, the setting may distract you. Perhaps there's too much light and all you can think about is how your body looks. Perhaps the bed, floor, or ground you're lying on is uncomfortable. Maybe you're worried that someone will come in. As you should know by now, worrying *about* something (anything!) during sex is not recommended if you want to feel highly aroused and have an orgasm.

Sometimes it's the lovemaking style of a partner that seems to put us off. You may have a new partner whose style is quite different from your own. Perhaps you like to start sex nice and slowly, with a lot of romantic talk, but your partner may enjoy clowning around first, or may begin by touching your clitoris. In each of these examples, there's an obvious difference between what you each like in order to get aroused, and this could easily lead to your feelings coming to a grinding halt.

Here are a few examples of how our conditions for arousal can be upset:

- You like lots of kissing. Your partner doesn't.
- You like having your back stroked. Your partner hasn't even found your back yet.
- You like to talk out your fantasies. Your partner thinks you're weird.
- You like to masturbate without anyone else in the house. The relatives have come to stay for two months.

- You're fairly conservative. Your partner likes sex toys and flimsy lingerie.
- You need to develop trust before having sex. Your new partner wants to have sex on your second date.

Can you see now how an understanding of your arousal pattern is the first step to working on your orgasm difficulties?

&

YOU MAY WANT to stop for a moment and think about how your turn-on/turn-off patterns developed. To do this, you need to focus on what you learned in the areas of sexuality and sexual relationships from:

- your parents, your grandparents (or those who raised you)
- your neighborhood
- your religion
- your school, your teachers
- your special relationships (boyfriends/girlfriends, lovers, long-term partners, husbands)
- life experiences.

**Now, let me give you a hint:** just because your parents didn't sit down and actually talk to you about sex doesn't mean you didn't receive a bundle of messages about your sexuality! It's the things that *aren't* said and the subtle *non-verbal* gestures, such as switching TV channels when a sexual topic appears, that teach us so well. Unfortunately, what we learn is more often negative than positive.

Now, let me take you one step further in understanding your sexual arousal patterns. Try the exercise on the next page. It will help you to understand your *orgasm patterns.*

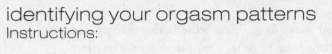

## identifying your orgasm patterns
### Instructions:

Make a list of situations, activities and types of people that are linked with **having an orgasm**. Also make a list of situations, activities and types of people that are linked with **not having an orgasm**.

|  | ORGASM | NO ORGASM |
|---|---|---|
| Sexual situations (Where/When you have sex) |  |  |
| Sexual activities (What you do sexually) |  |  |
| Types of people (Who you have sex with) |  |  |

Once again, take the time to sit and study your answers.

Are you surprised at what you found out about yourself? This exercise should have pinpointed more clearly the pattern behind your lack of orgasms. For some of you, understanding this picture will now suggest possible explanations for your orgasm difficulties. For others it may not be so clear.

Here are some of the more common patterns for women who orgasm at some times and not others:

### Sexual Situations
- unable to orgasm in any room except the bedroom
- unable to orgasm when other people are in the house
- unable to orgasm in the mornings before going to work

### Sexual Activities
- unable to orgasm during intercourse

- unable to orgasm without using a vibrator
- unable to orgasm without very hard pressure
- unable to orgasm when touched by a partner

**Types of People**
- unable to orgasm with a long-term partner or husband
- unable to orgasm with a new partner

Although there are many different patterns, the causes of most of them, fortunately, can be narrowed down to a small group of factors, as listed below:

## causes of women's orgasm difficulties:
women who can orgasm at some times and not others

**Cause #18:** Resentment towards a partner
**Cause #19:** Boredom with a partner
**Cause #20:** Loss of physical attraction to a partner
**Cause #21:** Trying too hard to please a partner
**Cause #22:** Difficulty in showing sexual passion
**Cause #23:** Thinking intercourse is the only way
**Cause #24:** Conditioning by habits and fantasies
**Cause #25:** Sexually abusive experiences

# CAUSE #18: |
resentment towards a partner

I KNOW I said this back in chapter 1, but let me repeat it here. Resentment towards a partner makes it hard to get sexually aroused because it . . .

- *stops* us wanting to be *close*
- *stops* us feeling *relaxed*
- *stops* us wanting to spend *time* with a partner
- *stops* us feeling *happy*

- *stops* us wanting to *enjoy* our partner
- *stops* us wanting to *please* our partner
- *stops* us *thinking* clearly

I could go on, but I think I've made my point. Resentment is really anger that isn't expressed openly. We might not show it, but inside we're seething about whatever made us angry in the first place.

- *and then* we become bitter about the whole thing
- *and then* we stop thinking clearly about what's been going on and see only *our* viewpoint
- *and then* we start to feel sorry for the way we've been treated

And so it goes. Resentment is like quicksand. The more we stay in it, the more we get sucked down into a whirlpool of negativity.

You'd think the last thing anyone would do is have sex with a partner they feel resentful towards. Yet, women often find themselves doing just that. It may be to keep the peace with a partner. Perhaps they're hoping sex will fix the problem.

Unfortunately, having sex with someone you're feeling resentful towards is likely to create more problems than it fixes. For example, you'll probably be feeling quite distant from your partner. Hardly the right condition for you to get highly aroused, is it?

And if you *always* feel resentful towards your partner, there's not much chance that sex is *ever* going to be enjoyable or arousing enough for you to have an orgasm.

A woman once came to me whose partner had had an affair twelve months previously. Even though she'd decided to have another go at the relationship and still felt attracted to her partner, most of her time was spent feeling resentful about what had happened. During sex she would often think about her partner being with the other person. Naturally, she then became upset and distracted, and soon lost her feelings of sexual arousal. When I saw her, she hadn't had an orgasm with her partner for nearly a year.

There are many reasons for women becoming resentful to the point where it affects their ability to orgasm. It may be because their partner doesn't help with the housework, spends little time with them, is aggressive. . . .

---

What about a partner who doesn't seem to want to touch me the way I want? I've given up repeating myself, but boy, do I feel resentful about it!

---

I'm not surprised. Having a partner who is not a skilled lover, and who isn't interested in learning how to arouse you better, is another common cause of resentment in women.

It really doesn't matter what causes your resentment—the result is still the same. You'll be unable to let your sexual feelings build enough to be able to climax.

---

## RATING

HOW much influence do you think **resentment towards your partner** has had on your sexual feelings?

| Influence in the past: | Influence now: |
|---|---|
| ❒ A great deal | ❒ A great deal |
| ❒ Quite a lot | ❒ Quite a lot |
| ❒ Some | ❒ Some |
| ❒ A little | ❒ A little |
| ❒ None | ❒ None |

# CAUSE #19:
## boredom with a partner

I MENTIONED IN the previous chapter that some people stop having orgasms because life is dull and mundane, and this rubs off onto their sex lives.

However, there are some women who have rather interesting lives, but are simply bored with their partner. They orgasm easily on their own or even with another person, yet can't feel much of a sexual spark with their regular partner. Perhaps they don't have a lot in common with their partner any more.

If this fits your situation, you may try to avoid sex because you're not interested in getting close to your partner. Or, you may have sex because you enjoy the sensations, but find that it's getting harder and harder to orgasm as time goes on.

Another kind of boredom is felt by women who enjoy the company of their partner in nonsexual situations, but are bored with what they're doing during sex.

---

> Exactly right! I love her dearly, but we've been doing
> the same thing now for ten years.

---

In that case, sex probably stopped being exciting some time ago and is now routine

---

> . . . and predictable . . . and unexciting.

---

It's also predictable that if neither you nor your partner has made any attempts to spark things up a bit, orgasms are likely to be a thing of the past. Remember, you can't have an orgasm if you don't start climbing the arousal hill. And you can't start the climb if you're not interested or your sexual feelings aren't being triggered.

Interestingly, some women in this situation have no trouble having an orgasm during masturbation. How come? Well, they excite themselves by using fantasies from their Turn-On Lists. In other words, they select pictures of sexual scenes and partners that excite them. If a fantasy becomes boring, all they have to do is change it to something more interesting. A woman may even have orgasms in her sleep when a (nonboring) sexy story pops into her dreams.

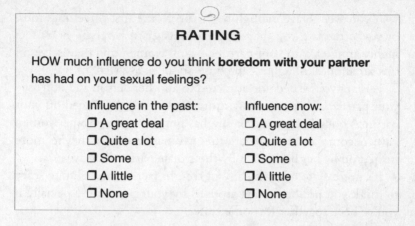

## RATING

HOW much influence do you think **boredom with your partner** has had on your sexual feelings?

Influence in the past:
- ❏ A great deal
- ❏ Quite a lot
- ❏ Some
- ❏ A little
- ❏ None

Influence now:
- ❏ A great deal
- ❏ Quite a lot
- ❏ Some
- ❏ A little
- ❏ None

# CAUSE #20:
## loss of physical attraction to a partner

IT'S A SAD fact, but some women find they're no longer attracted to their partners. They don't necessarily dislike them or find them boring. It's just that their body or manner doesn't arouse them sexually the way they used to.

If you feel this is true for you, check this out in the quiz below (be as honest with yourself as you can):

## physical attraction quiz

1. Do you like the look of your partner's body?  
   Yes ❏   No ❏

2. Does your partner's body fit the physical characteristics that turn you on (see Turn-On Lists)?  
   Yes ❏   No ❏

3. Are you happy with the way your partner grooms his or her body?  
   Yes ❏   No ❏

4. Are there any mannerisms your partner uses that you find a big turn-off?  
   Yes ❏   No ❏

If you were brave enough to say no to the first three questions, or yes to the last, you may have the answer to why you don't feel highly aroused with your partner. Many women find themselves in this situation, although it can come about in a variety of ways.

Perhaps you've become attracted to another person and don't see your partner as appealing any more. Perhaps you're turned off your partner's body because he or she has put on weight. Some women have become attracted to another woman and find they're more turned on by her body than by their male partner's body.

It's not easy to admit to any of this. In fact, it can be quite scary to think you no longer feel aroused by your partner—especially if you've been together for some time.

---

It sure is scary. I mean, what do I do now—fake it,
use fantasies to get turned on, or walk out?

---

Good question! It's going to depend on your particular situation. Some women want to stay in the relationship. So they feel okay about pretending to be aroused by their partner. Others just can't hide what they're really feeling. We don't often hear about it, but many women fantasize about someone else while making love with their partners; it helps them to get aroused and avoid accusations about not being interested in sex.

And, yes, some women leave the relationship because they can't do any of these things. Maybe they feel it's time to be with a partner who is attractive to them.

Oh, and there's one more question I should add to the previous quiz:

## physical attraction quiz
### (continued)

| | Yes | No |
|---|---|---|
| Have your feelings for your partner now changed, as a result of the loss of attraction, so that you see him or her as a companion or close friend rather than as a "lover"? | ☐ | ☐ |

If the answer to this question is yes, you may still see your partner as a good person for whom you care deeply. You can see how others would find him or her attractive. Perhaps you wish with all your heart that you could still feel attracted as you once did.

---

> But, I don't and that's just it! Something's changed inside me. We get on well. Yet, I feel more like a sister than a lover.

---

Which makes it impossible to enjoy sex, doesn't it? It doesn't matter how good-looking or well groomed your partner is. None of this will count if you don't feel the kind of attraction that lets your arousal build to orgasm.

---

## RATING

HOW much influence do you think **loss of physical attraction to your partner** has had on your sexual feelings?

| Influence in the past: | Influence now: |
|---|---|
| ❑ A great deal | ❑ A great deal |
| ❑ Quite a lot | ❑ Quite a lot |
| ❑ Some | ❑ Some |
| ❑ A little | ❑ A little |
| ❑ None | ❑ None |

---

# CAUSE #21:
## trying too hard to please a partner

SOME WOMEN CAN orgasm on their own during masturbation, but just can't get aroused enough to climax with a partner. Does this seem to describe you? Then you may find that even though you enjoy being with your partner, it doesn't stop you from getting stuck on a plateau or diving into a valley, instead of heading up the arousal hill.

> That's right. And if you think I'm going to tell my
> partner that it's easier on my own, forget it!

That's all right, although I think it's better if you can talk to a partner about sexual difficulties. However, I know that some partners react, either by thinking it's their fault or by telling *you* it's your problem. I doubt that you're going to feel good with either of these reactions.

Of course, there may be something your partner is doing that is a turn-off for you. Check this out. If there doesn't seem to be anything you can identify, it may be something *you're* doing during sex that makes orgasm difficult.

A very common cause of orgasm difficulties in women who can orgasm at some times and not others is *worrying too much about a partner's needs and expectations* during sex.

Women have often been taught to pay special attention to the needs of others (such as their children, partner, and parents). Unfortunately, this teaching follows them into the bedroom. Instead of relaxing and enjoying what's happening in their own body, all attention becomes focused on making their partner happy. Before long, they become a sexual *spectator* rather than participant. They're *thinking about what they're doing,* rather than just doing what feels pleasurable.

> So true! I put a lot of effort into making love to
> my partner, but can't seem to relax if the
> same thing is being done to me.

Well, if you think about it, making love with another person is quite complicated. We have to focus not only on our partner's needs, arousal and bodily reactions, but also on our own as well.

You may find this hard to do because your upbringing has taught you to concentrate on the *other* person, not yourself. Having the focus on you may feel "wrong" or uncomfortable, simply because this goes against everything you've learned.

**To be able to orgasm, however, you need to feel comfortable about having the attention on *you*.**

If you think only of your partner, I'm afraid there's little chance you'll be able to build your sexual arousal high enough to orgasm. This is not to say you shouldn't try and please your partner sexually. But there has to be a balance.

**Good sex is about both *giving* and *receiving* pleasure.**

For most of us this is easier to do when we're masturbating on our own than when with a partner, because we only have one person to satisfy: ourselves.

☙

NOW, LET ME give you another version of "trying too hard to please a partner" that is also common among women.

Do you worry about whether your partner approves of you or not? Do you carry this worry into your sexual activity? Then there's a good chance orgasm will be hard to reach. Concern about what our partners think of us is another way in which women focus too much on them.

During sex, you may have negative thoughts like those below:

- *Does he or she like me?*
- *Am I doing the right thing?*
- *Am I touching in the right place?*
- *Am I attractive enough?*

---

You've forgotten, "Am I a better lover than the ex-partner?" From experience I can tell you, this thought's a real dampener on sexual feelings.

---

Are you surprised? We could also add,

- *Have I put on too much weight?*
- *Will I look funny if I orgasm?*
- *Is it okay to show I enjoy sex?*

Sound familiar? Then it may be that fear of your partner's disapproval is stopping you from losing yourself in the sexual situation. If this is the case, you'll find it easier to have orgasms on your own or with someone whose opinion you don't care about. It's a different story when you're with someone you want to impress. You'll be so busy worrying about your partner's reactions and thinking negatively about yourself that you'll forget to enjoy your own sexuality.

You become the spectator *par excellence* (translation: the best there is!). Not only are you standing on the sidelines watching the whole show, you're also *judging* whether you rate a "pass" or "fail." And if you mostly rate as a failure, your arousal will head in only one direction, dear reader: all the way *down* the arousal hill (and it will be a fast slide to the bottom, I can tell you!). I call it **orgasmic meltdown.**

---

### RATING

HOW much influence do you think **trying too hard to please a partner** has had on your sexual feelings?

| Influence in the past: | Influence now: |
| --- | --- |
| ❏ A great deal | ❏ A great deal |
| ❏ Quite a lot | ❏ Quite a lot |
| ❏ Some | ❏ Some |
| ❏ A little | ❏ A little |
| ❏ None | ❏ None |

## CAUSE #22:
### difficulty in showing sexual passion

SOME WOMEN WHO can orgasm at some times and not others find themselves consciously holding back their sexual feelings in *some* sexual situations, during *some* sexual activities or with *some* partners. Instead of letting their arousal become stronger, they cut it off or keep it at low levels, so that orgasm simply can't occur.

There are many ways in which women find it difficult to show sexual feelings. For example, you may feel awkward about showing sexual passion in front of a *new* partner. Or, maybe you can't let yourself go when involved in sexual activities that you've been taught are wrong or dirty (e.g., masturbation, group sex, sex before marriage, oral sex). Some women get worried that if they *really* let their sexual feelings out, they will say or do something embarrassing.

Sometimes the problem is showing passion to an *old* rather than a new partner. I often see women who entered marriage or a long-term relationship when very young. In the early part of the relationship, they lacked confidence and were unsure of themselves sexually. But, as they matured, they developed the confidence to express their sexual passion in a more positive way. And they wanted a mature sexual relationship to match.

Problems arise, however, if they continue to make love in the old way. You know, just as they did when she was young, shy and inexperienced. This makes it hard for her to express her new passionate self and can lead to feelings of frustration. Unfortunately, many women are nervous about asking for something different.

---

That's exactly my story. How do I tell my partner that I've become more passionate? I'm ready to be less inhibited and more sexy, but I don't want to be thought of as some kind of sex maniac.

---

Join the club (the Secretly Sexy Club). Like you, many women start to feel much sexier *inside* as they get older, but are afraid to tell their partner. If you've been seen in bed as sensible, quiet, rational, unassertive, demure, easygoing, controlled, unemotional, or not particularly interested, it can be scary to consider showing another side to your character.

And, if your partner seems to be threatened by ways in which you're changing outside the bedroom, you'll probably find it impossible to show him or her the "new sexual you." Understandably, you're going to feel resentful and stressed as you pretend to be someone you're not.

Other emotions can also play a part in making women hold back sexually: shyness or nervousness about having sex with a new partner; embarrassment about trying oral sex for the first time; fear of not living up to a partner's expectations; anxiety about enjoying sexual passion without a partner. These are just some examples, but I'm sure you can think of others.

Now, how easy do you think it is to get turned on with these kinds of emotions churning around inside? I can assure you, it's not easy at all. Shyness, nervousness, resentment and similar emotions lead to anxiety and tension—not the relaxation and enjoyment that is needed for you to become aroused enough to orgasm. It's highly unlikely that you'll be *swooning with unbridled passion that is crying out for release,* as the romance novels phrase it.

But I'm sure you already know this!

---

### RATING

HOW much influence do you think **difficulty in showing sexual passion** has had on your sexual feelings?

| Influence in the past: | Influence now: |
| --- | --- |
| ❒ A great deal | ❒ A great deal |
| ❒ Quite a lot | ❒ Quite a lot |
| ❒ Some | ❒ Some |
| ❒ A little | ❒ A little |
| ❒ None | ❒ None |

---

## CAUSE #23:
### thinking intercourse is the only way

IT'S AMAZING HOW often I hear women say they can't orgasm, only to find that actually they *can* orgasm quite easily during sexual activity involving oral, manual, or body contact sex. What they mean is *they can't orgasm during vaginal intercourse.*

Of course, by saying, *I can't orgasm,* they make themselves feel like failures, when the truth is that they're very accomplished sexually.

Unfortunately, vaginal intercourse is often presented as *real* sex, or the only *true* way of being sexual. All other forms of sex are then seen as secondary or *foreplay.* As a result, any orgasm reached during "foreplay" is not considered to be a "proper" orgasm.

Personally I'd like to *ban* the word *foreplay*, because it suggests that only vaginal intercourse is sex and anything else is . . . well, fooling around—*which just isn't true.*

There's great pressure on heterosexual (male/female) couples to practice sex in the so-called *right* way. Anyone who reads romance novels or watches Hollywood movies has learned what the "right" way is supposed to be: vaginal intercourse that leads to earth-shattering orgasms simultaneously felt by both people. Anything else is seen as second rate.

This message is so widespread that it's not surprising many women believe that sex is not "good sex" unless they orgasm during intercourse.

Of course, you may want to orgasm during intercourse *for your own enjoyment,* not because it's the "proper" thing to do. I'll be discussing in chapter 10 how you might be able to do this.

Perhaps, however, it's your partner who thinks there's something wrong with not being able to orgasm during intercourse. You yourself may not care whether you climax during intercourse or not, but it's your partner who wants this, and you feel pressured to oblige. Don't forget that men have also been taught the same message (even if they haven't read the romantic novels).

If this fits your situation, the difference between your sexual wishes and those of your partner is the problem, not your difficulty in having an orgasm. If you prefer to orgasm with oral sex rather than intercourse, then that's perfectly okay.

---

But I thought everyone who was "sexually mature"
could orgasm with a partner during intercourse. Isn't
this what I'm trying to achieve?

---

Oh, dear, now you're sounding like one of those outdated text-books on sex that I can only hope are gathering dust in the basements of libraries. I prefer to describe sexual maturity as

**. . . being able to fully enjoy your sexuality in any way that makes you feel fulfilled, safe, and respected.**

**This may or may not include sexual intercourse.**

The important thing to remember is that if you feel pressured into trying to have orgasms during intercourse, you most definitely *won't* have them. The negative thought, *There must be something wrong with me because I can't orgasm during intercourse,* will act as a turn-off and dampen your arousal.

Now, I may be wrong, but the idea that you should have an orgasm during intercourse sounds like a goal you've set for yourself. Remember my words in chapter 1 about becoming goal-focused during sex. It's a sure way to stop yourself relaxing and enjoying the moment—another clear path to orgasmic meltdown.

Q

BEFORE WE GO any further, I think I need to mention a few facts about intercourse. Firstly, *many* women do *not* have orgasms during intercourse. Secondly, many women don't worry or care about having orgasms during vaginal intercourse and enjoy climaxing in other ways. Oral sex is often rated as the most preferred and easiest way of reaching orgasm.

Thirdly, intercourse is not the easiest way for women to orgasm. Some intercourse positions don't allow male and female bodies to fit together well enough for the glans and shaft of the clitoris to be touched directly. Because of this, it may be difficult to stay highly aroused once you begin intercourse.

And fourthly, it's a myth that if you and your partner are well matched and love each other, orgasms should happen easily and naturally during intercourse (or, for that matter, during any sexual activity).

Having orgasms during intercourse has a lot to do with the positions you use, how sensitive the internal parts of your clitoris become during arousal, how turned on you are before intercourse takes place, whether you also use other forms of touch while having intercourse, how safe and intimate you feel with your partner, how important intercourse is to you, and so on.

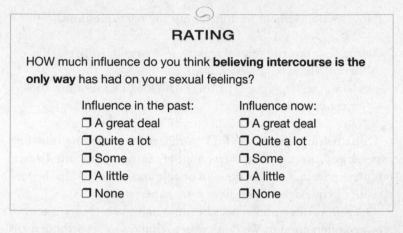

**RATING**

HOW much influence do you think **believing intercourse is the only way** has had on your sexual feelings?

| Influence in the past: | Influence now: |
|---|---|
| ❒ A great deal | ❒ A great deal |
| ❒ Quite a lot | ❒ Quite a lot |
| ❒ Some | ❒ Some |
| ❒ A little | ❒ A little |
| ❒ None | ❒ None |

## CAUSE #24:
### conditioning by habits and fantasies

PAST SEXUAL EXPERIENCES, especially our first, can have a powerful influence on how we react sexually *now*. Try the following exercise and see if you learn anything about yourself.

## how past sexual experiences can affect our sexual reactions
think back to your:

- first date
- first experiences of sexual arousal
- first orgasm
- first romantic moment
- most exciting sexual moment as a young person
- clearest early sexual memory

Shut your eyes and picture each scene as clearly as you can. Try to recall the colors, the smells, your surroundings. If possible, remember the reactions you had: your feelings and your thoughts.

Now, take a moment to think about my next questions.

- Are your favorite ways of making love or climaxing *now* similar to what you did back *then?*
- Do you tend to choose partners who look like your first date or romantic love?

Don't be surprised if you find a similarity. It's amazing how first experiences can stay with us (even if they weren't pleasant). In fact, our preferences for certain types of people and certain sexual behaviors are often learned from these early experiences.

Over time, these preferences become habits, especially if they're repeated often enough. We don't stop to think why something turns us on or why we like having sex in a certain way—we just know this is part of who we are and what we like.

Sometimes our sexual habits can stop our arousal from building to orgasm. For example, if you have difficulty climaxing when a partner is touching you gently, it may be that you've learned over time to prefer a firmer touch. Perhaps you've always masturbated (and had an orgasm) using a firm pressure, and this habit has taught you to enjoy a strong touch, rather than gentle stroking.

If you're not getting the touch that really arouses you, it may be hard to relax and let your sexual pleasure build to orgasm. Instead, you'll lie there getting annoyed that your partner can't touch you in the "right" way, or worse still, blaming yourself for not being able to orgasm.

Some women have great difficulty becoming highly aroused with a partner because of the way they masturbate. Some styles of masturbating aren't easily copied by a partner. For example, you may have always had an orgasm while lying on your stomach, *or.* squeezing your legs together (perhaps with a pillow in between), *or* sitting *or* kneeling. Because you've always masturbated this way, your sexual feelings have been conditioned to build more strongly *only* in these positions. When you try another position with a partner, it's likely to feel strange and uncomfortable and stop you from getting in the mood for having an orgasm.

---

Well, I had my first orgasm on my own at the age of
thirty-eight, using a vibrator. It was great, but now I
can't orgasm except with the vibrator. This is
probably one of those habits you're talking about,
because I kind of feel hooked on it.

---

You may indeed be "hooked" on your vibrator, especially if you're not prepared to try other ways of getting aroused. You've *taught* your body to get aroused in this way. Of course, there's nothing wrong with being able to orgasm only with a vibrator—unless you also want to be able to orgasm without it.

Other sexual habits can also make it difficult to orgasm. I've spoken to many women who prefer to lie very still during sex. Orgasm is often hard work, and they feel the only way to get there is by concentrating on what they're doing. If they have to move or speak during sex with a partner (or even on their own), they get turned off (and more than a little annoyed, in some cases).

For some women, the need to lie still in order to orgasm is caused by the tug-of-war between negative thoughts and pleasurable stroking that I mentioned in chapter 3. But for others, it can be a learned pattern, usually begun in teenage years, when trying to masturbate quietly so the rest of the family wouldn't hear.

Once again, this style isn't necessarily a problem unless you want to be able to orgasm in a different way.

What this all means is that sexual arousal patterns can be learned. Any sexual activity, thought, fantasy, type of person, or situation that arouses you sexually will become a part of your Turn-On List *if used or repeated often enough.*

Doing something occasionally is unlikely to condition your sexual arousal (but see Cause # 25). Generally, you have to repeat it over and over. The more you repeat it, the stronger the learning.

Sometimes this can cause problems with orgasm. Let me explain, using the example of sexual fantasies.

Fantasies can be very powerful ways of conditioning our sexual arousal. If you use the same fantasy over and over, you'll find yourself becoming aroused more easily when you use it, *or* have sex with someone who fits it, *or* do something similar to it.

Eventually, however, (and this is the interesting bit) you might find yourself unable to get aroused at all *unless* everything fits the fantasy exactly. Your arousal and orgasms will become linked so strongly to the fantasy that nothing else will give you the same level of pleasure.

I once counseled a woman who only ever fantasized about being raped. In her first sexual experience she had been pressured to have sex by her boyfriend. He had been rough and uncaring but, nevertheless, she had become aroused and had an orgasm, the novelty and touch probably triggering her reactions. From then on, whenever she masturbated, she always pictured being taken by force. And she always had an orgasm easily.

Her problems began when she became involved with a gentle, caring man. Although she adored him, she simply could not orgasm with him. Her arousal pattern was by this time so strongly linked with rough sex that she could not switch to a different way of being aroused.

Take some time, then, to think over the orgasm pattern you identified earlier in this chapter. It may be that you've learned to orgasm in some ways and not others because of certain fantasies and habits.

---

## RATING

HOW much influence do you think **conditioning by habits and fantasies** has had on your sexual feelings?

| Influence in the past: | Influence now: |
| --- | --- |
| ❏ A great deal | ❏ A great deal |
| ❏ Quite a lot | ❏ Quite a lot |
| ❏ Some | ❏ Some |
| ❏ A little | ❏ A little |
| ❏ None | ❏ None |

# CAUSE #25:
## sexually abusive experiences

ABUSIVE EXPERIENCES MAY interfere with our enjoyment of sex on some occasions and not others. For example, if the sexual abuse you experienced in childhood or adulthood involved oral sex, you may now have trouble enjoying oral sex, because it reminds you of what you were forced to do during the times of abuse.

Or you may have difficulty feeling aroused with anyone who is dark-haired, if the person who sexually abused you was dark-haired. And so on. There can be all kinds of reminders of those abusive experiences. Some will affect sexual arousal and orgasm. Others may not.

If you've been sexually abused, you may find that sex with a partner doesn't feel safe, and you're only able to have an orgasm on your own. Or you may have realized that certain sexual activities or positions make you anxious (e.g., lying under your partner) and must be avoided if you want to build your arousal and orgasm.

Some women have discovered that it's easier to let themselves become sexually aroused with a woman because a male partner reminds them of their attacker.

I've known women who were happily sexual and orgasmic with partners *until* they began to think seriously about past abusive experiences. After being reminded of their earlier experiences in this way, they found that during sex they would confuse their partner with the person who originally attacked them. Naturally, this left them feeling tense and anxious, and unable to become aroused enough to orgasm. Again, masturbation is often the only way they can safely let their arousal build.

---

## RATING

HOW much influence do you think **sexually abusive experiences** have had on your sexual feelings?

| Influence in the past: | Influence now: |
| --- | --- |
| ❐ A great deal | ❐ A great deal |
| ❐ Quite a lot | ❐ Quite a lot |
| ❐ Some | ❐ Some |
| ❐ A little | ❐ A little |
| ❐ None | ❐ None |

---

# conclusions |

BEING ABLE TO orgasm at some times and not others can be confusing and frustrating. Hopefully, this chapter has helped you to understand your arousal and orgasm patterns and to recognise possible causes of your difficulties. As you can see, none of the causes I've outlined are weird or mysterious. In fact, they're the sorts of things many of us experience from time to time.

The next step is to decide if you want to change what's happening in your life so that you can orgasm at all times. Remember, any change must be made because it seems *right* for you. Making changes just to please someone else is a nice thought but, as I've said before, unlikely to lead to success.

# where do I go from here?
## making changes

Well here we are, ready to talk about *change*. So far, you've put your energy into understanding what it is that's making orgasm difficult for you. Now comes the interesting part—what you can do to make orgasm happen more easily.

---

Great! But from what I've now learned,
it could take years to sort myself out.

---

Maybe not. Unless there's something completely out of your control, it's probably going to take less time than you think. For some, it will be a few months; for others, longer.

So, just relax. You've come this far, what does it matter if you take the next six months going through the suggestions and Change Programs I'm offering? Don't start pressuring yourself with another goal to strive for (you know what I mean: the *I-want-an-orgasm-and-I-want-it-soon* goal).

**The only goal you should have is the goal to try the ideas I put forward in the next few chapters.**

You don't even have to be absolutely certain they'll work. That would be asking too much, especially if you've tried programs before and nothing changed.

All you need is bit of good old-fashioned *motivation*. By this I mean, you need to:

- be determined to do your best
- be prepared to put in some effort to try the suggestions or exercises I offer
- be interested enough to *think* about what's going on
- have the desire to make changes for *yourself*
- be open to new ideas and feelings
- be patient—nothing's going to happen overnight

I'm sure some of you will be keen to make changes now that the likely causes of your orgasm difficulties have been identified. I also realize, however, that some of you may be feeling rather daunted by the thought of taking the next few steps.

---

Hey, what if I try your suggestions
and I still can't orgasm?

---

Many women have the same fear at this point. And it's completely understandable. All I can do is help you reduce the chance of this happening. The best way to do that is to outline the conditions likely to make my suggestions and Change Programs work. I've listed these conditions below. Place a check next to those that exist for you at the moment.

**From yourself:**
- ❏ a strong wish that the suggestions and Programs will help you to orgasm
- ❏ a readiness to reorganize your life so there's enough time to carry out the suggestions and do the set exercises properly

❏ a desire to become fully comfortable with your sexual arousal and to enjoy it

❏ a willingness to consider changing aspects of your lifestyle that interfere with your sexual arousal

❏ a willingness to develop attitudes towards sexuality that may differ from those of your parents

If you want to be able to orgasm with a partner, you also need the following:

**From a relationship:**
❏ a supportive and enthusiastic partner

❏ a willingness to talk with your partner about how you're feeling and thinking while carrying out the suggestions and doing the Change Programs

❏ feelings of love and caring for your partner

❏ a wish to be sexual and have an orgasm with your partner

If these conditions exist, and you follow the ideas outlined in the next few chapters, you stand a good chance of being able to orgasm more easily. *But note:* each condition that is missing will make things that much harder. Sometimes it's better to wait until all the elements are in place.

However, just as there are many different causes of women's orgasm difficulties, there are also many different ways in which changes can be made. In fact, I've had to use *seven* chapters to cover these. I'd be surprised if you couldn't find something to start on, no matter how small. You don't have to tackle the bigger picture just yet. And you don't have to change everything at this very moment. Take your time, do what you can and be patient about the rest.

So read through the chapters that apply to the causes of your type of orgasm difficulty and see if there's something that you can work on. If you decide this isn't the time, then put this book down and come back to it when you're ready. You could also get some help from a professional therapist, such as a psychologist, about the conditions that are missing.

# what needs changing?

HOPEFULLY, THE CAUSES of your difficulties with orgasm will now be clearer to you. If you're still unsure, you may like to wait for a few days and then reread the previous chapters. A second reading may help. If not, try to find someone trained in sexual therapy who can take you through the relevant sections. Sometimes another point of view can assist you to look at things differently.

Before we go on to *how* to change, let's summarize *what* needs changing. In the previous three chapters, I asked you to rate the effect of each of the twenty-five causes on you, both at present and in the past.

Take a few moments now to transfer this information to the chart on the next page (if using a library copy, write it into your notebook). The page numbers for each rating scale are listed in the chart. To help your understanding, I've divided the causes into five headings: *lifestyle, personal, health, sexual, relationships.*

Transfer the X from each rating scale onto the chart. Here's an example of what to do:

| Lifestyle | | great deal | quite a lot | some | a little | none |
|---|---|---|---|---|---|---|
| **Cause #1:** Being a busy person (page 56) | Influence NOW | X | | | | |
| | PAST Influence | | | | X | |
| **Cause #13:** Life became full of stress and upset (page 85) | Influence NOW | X | | | | |
| | PAST Influence | | | | X | |

# causes of orgasm difficulties
## Summary of past and present influence

| Lifestyle | | great deal | quite a lot | some | a little | none |
|---|---|---|---|---|---|---|
| **Cause #1:** Being a busy person (page 56) | Influence NOW | | | | | |
| | PAST Influence | | | | | |
| **Cause #13:** Life became full of stress and upset (page 85) | Influence NOW | | | | | |
| | PAST Influence | | | | | |
| **Cause #14:** Life became boring (page 90) | Influence NOW | | | | | |
| | PAST Influence | | | | | |
| **Cause #15:** Less time taken to become aroused (page 93) | Influence NOW | | | | | |
| | PAST Influence | | | | | |
| **Personal** | | | | | | |
| **Cause #2:** Being goal-focused (page 58) | Influence NOW | | | | | |
| | PAST Influence | | | | | |
| **Cause #3:** Needing to stay in control of emotions (page 61) | Influence NOW | | | | | |
| | PAST Influence | | | | | |
| **Cause #8:** Feeling guilty about enjoying yourself (page 75) | Influence NOW | | | | | |
| | PAST Influence | | | | | |
| **Cause #9:** Feeling guilty because of childhood sex (page 77) | Influence NOW | | | | | |
| | PAST Influence | | | | | |
| **Cause #21:** Trying too hard to please a partner (page 121) | Influence NOW | | | | | |
| | PAST Influence | | | | | |
| **Cause #22:** Difficulty showing sexual passion (page 124) | Influence NOW | | | | | |
| | PAST Influence | | | | | |

| Health | | great deal | quite a lot | some | a little | none |
|---|---|---|---|---|---|---|
| **Cause #11:** Long-term use of some medications (page 79) | Influence NOW | | | | | |
| | PAST Influence | | | | | |
| **Cause #12:** Physical conditions (page 80) | Influence NOW | | | | | |
| | PAST Influence | | | | | |
| **Cause #16:** Sex became painful (page 94) | Influence NOW | | | | | |
| | PAST Influence | | | | | |
| **Cause #17:** Changes to health (page 98) | Influence NOW | | | | | |
| | PAST Influence | | | | | |

## Sexual

| | | great deal | quite a lot | some | a little | none |
|---|---|---|---|---|---|---|
| **Cause #4:** Lacking enough information about sexual arousal (page 65) | Influence NOW | | | | | |
| | PAST Influence | | | | | |
| **Cause #6:** Not enough time to become highly aroused (page 71) | Influence NOW | | | | | |
| | PAST Influence | | | | | |
| **Cause #7:** Some fantasies can affect arousal (page 73) | Influence NOW | | | | | |
| | PAST Influence | | | | | |
| **Cause #10:** Past sexual abuse (page 78) | Influence NOW | | | | | |
| | PAST Influence | | | | | |
| **Cause #23:** Thinking intercouse is the only way (page 126) | Influence NOW | | | | | |
| | PAST Influence | | | | | |
| **Cause #24:** Conditioning by habits and fantasies (page 129) | Influence NOW | | | | | |
| | PAST Influence | | | | | |
| **Cause #25:** Sexually abusive experiences (page 133) | Influence NOW | | | | | |
| | PAST Influence | | | | | |

| Relationships | | great deal | quite a lot | some | a little | none |
|---|---|---|---|---|---|---|
| **Cause #5:** Unable to communicate sexual needs (page 70) | Influence NOW | | | | | |
| | PAST Influence | | | | | |
| **Cause #18:** Resentment towards a partner (page 115) | Influence NOW | | | | | |
| | PAST Influence | | | | | |
| **Cause #19:** Boredom with a partner (page 117) | Influence NOW | | | | | |
| | PAST Influence | | | | | |
| **Cause #20:** Loss of physical attraction to a partner (page 119) | Influence NOW | | | | | |
| | PAST Influence | | | | | |

**Comments:**

Now study the chart. What does it tell you about your situation?

---

Heavens, was this such a good idea? Just about
everything seems to be affecting me! I didn't know I
was this complicated.

---

Now just relax. We're *all* complicated. I rarely counsel a women
with a simple, neat background to her sexual difficulties. Just remember, the more you understand yourself, the more exact you can be
in targeting the problem areas. Try to see the chart as a good chance
to get the whole picture.

Let's take it bit by bit.

## FIRST STEP

1. Look only at the two headings, Great Deal (of influence) and
   Quite a Lot (of influence).

2. Under these headings, look at where you put your crosses in each area: Lifestyle, Personal, Health, Sexual, and Relationships.

Can you find a pattern in the information?

3. Do the causes of your orgasm difficulties seem to fit into one of these areas more than the others, or are they spread across the board?
4. Within each area, are there several causes that seem to be affecting you? Or is there just one that seems to account for your orgasm difficulties?

It may help to write down your findings.

## SECOND STEP

1. Still concentrating only on the two headings, Great Deal (of influence) and Quite a Lot (of influence), look at the crosses next to the heading, Influence NOW.
2. Then compare this with the causes that were *PAST Influences*. Has anything changed?
3. You may now want to try to work out which of the causes seem to have been early influences *pushing* you in the direction of your orgasm difficulties, which causes seemed to *start off* your difficulties, and which seem to be *keeping* the problem going.

It's not always easy to sort out the differences between these three sets of causes, so don't worry if you're not sure. If you need help, a professional therapist will be able to guide you.

As you can see, change does not always mean doing something different in the bedroom. It might also mean rethinking how your life is organized, or how you personally approach issues. It may require different ways of adapting to health issues or reexamining what you want from your relationship.

In the next few chapters I'll talk about these five areas and the changes you can make in each so as to experience higher levels of sexual arousal. For some of you, tackling the cause will be enough to allow you to feel more highly aroused and to orgasm.

On the other hand, for many of you, this may be just the beginning. Even after you've made changes to your attitudes, behavior or lifestyle, it can still be difficult to take that first step towards actually doing something sexual. After months and sometimes years (a lifetime, perhaps) of being unable to orgasm, it's not always easy to just let yourself go sexually. Most women tend to feel self-conscious and awkward.

---

Hey, it's also going to be hard to let go with my partner. I'm going to feel like a schoolgirl out on her first date. It's silly after all these years together, but that's how I feel.

---

Actually, you've described exactly how many women feel. To help you through your awkwardness, I'll be outlining two Programs especially for this purpose:

- **The Personal Change Program** (chapter 13): designed to help you feel comfortable with being highly aroused and experiencing orgasms on your own.
- **The Couple Change Program** (chapter 14): for those of you currently in a relationship and wanting to experience orgasms with your partner.

Both Programs can help you to enjoy sexual feelings (again?) in a positive and relaxing way. Even more importantly, they can move you over the hump of feeling aroused to a certain point and then cutting off.

No matter what the cause of your orgasm difficulties, no matter how positive you're now feeling, no matter how supportive your partner is

**. . . continually getting sexually aroused to a certain level and no further will teach (condition) your body and mind to react sexually** *only* **in this way.**

By now, you've probably been conditioned into a start-stop pattern:

**Start to get aroused . . . reach a certain point . . . switch off.**

And it will happen so fast you won't even realize you've switched off until it's too late. The Personal Change Program and Couple Change Program will help you to undo this "switching-off" habit.

**A gentle warning, though:** the aim of these Programs is to help you orgasm easily. This does not mean you will necessarily orgasm *every time*. Be realistic.

Remember, there are so many things that can affect women's sexual arousal. We can all have difficulty with orgasm at some time or another.

What's more important is for you to develop *confidence* in your ability to orgasm. You can do this: firstly by understanding what causes your orgasm difficulty; and secondly, by learning what changes you can realistically make that will help you to get aroused enough to orgasm.

Knowing what's going on and what you can do about it is a good start to feeling confident. Of course, you also have to *make* those changes.

I recommend you read through all of the remaining chapters. Don't skip sections unless they are completely irrelevant to the causes of your orgasm difficulty.

I also *strongly* recommend you do the Personal Change Program before the Couple Change Program. It's much easier making sexual changes on your own, since you don't have to worry about your partner's expectations. I know some of you may not want to do it this way, but I'd still recommend you read chapter 13. There are many useful tidbits of information that can help you.

---

I just wish there was a pill I could take. It would be
so much easier—and quicker.

---

If only it were that simple! It's true that for some women with physical changes there can be medications and even certain devices that help to overcome the effects of their medical condition (see chapter 12). But there isn't a pill that will change negative thinking or attitudes. And no drug or device will mend a poor relationship, remove feelings of resentment or change sexual habits.

To put it simply, you'll probably have to make the changes yourself. Interestingly, many women who do so feel pleased that they *have* done it themselves.

# 8

# making
# lifestyle
# changes

For many women, changing the way they go about their daily lives is the key to reaching orgasm more easily. This is not as difficult as you might think.

## being a busy person |

YOU KNOW YOU have to stop being so busy. You don't need me to tell you. Yet, we both know how hard it is to rid yourself of lifestyle pressures.

---

You're right. I KNOW I'm too busy. AND too stressed. But there doesn't seem to be much I can do about it. My job's hectic and now my mother's ill.

---

Yes, there's always a real-life situation we have to deal with. Unfortunately, these pressures play a big part in your orgasm difficulties. What to do? Give up wanting to have your sexual needs met? I hope not.

The most obvious change (and one that works for many women) is to take some time for yourself before going to bed. Don't keep yourself busy until the time you're ready to collapse into bed with exhaustion. Deliberately stop doing chores so that you leave time to unwind (even thirty minutes will be enough). When you head off for bed, do so with the idea that you're going to enjoy a few minutes relaxing, dreaming, or cuddling and talking in bed with your partner. Concentrate on feeling peaceful and quiet. Get yourself in a mood so that if lovemaking begins to happen, you'll be more relaxed and more likely to enjoy it.

The same advice applies to those of you who don't have a partner. Why wait until you're ready to go to sleep before heading off to bed? Instead, slow down earlier in the evening. Relax with a book, music, or some television. Concentrate on switching off your thinking from your busy schedule. Think about how enjoyable it would be to masturbate while relaxing in bed.

In other words, give yourself a chance to turn your thinking off from the day. You need time to change from being a career woman, dutiful daughter, wife, and mother to being a woman with sexual desires.

It's also important to take some time to relax on the weekends. Now, before you groan loudly, I'm not talking hours and hours of relaxation here. Even thirty minutes of slowing down can be enough to change your focus from what you've called things-that-just-have-to-be-done and onto *you*. Change your attitude to lying in bed. Make it time for yourself, rather than "wasting time." And don't forget that sex is one way of taking time for yourself and relaxing.

Have you noticed how there's always *another* job that has to be done? No matter how hard you work to get through the list you made yesterday, there'll always be more things to add to it today— and tomorrow. Don't you feel like one of those little mice running around a wheel? The more you run, the faster everything gets, until you collapse exhausted (and, more than likely, sick).

> Hey, I'm really struggling with this. If I don't get
> everything on my list finished, I feel I'm a failure.

You're not alone in thinking like that, believe me! Most women have been taught to be superwomen, able to do everything and do it perfectly. There's just one problem. Being superwoman *and* highly aroused don't go together very well.

So, it's time to decide whether this pressured lifestyle is the way you want to live. Remember, all I'm suggesting is that you take a little time to unwind and remind yourself that you are also a woman with needs: sexual needs, intimacy needs, fun needs.

**Give your sexual needs and feelings a place of importance in your life.**

Don't make them a last priority, as many women with orgasm difficulties do. Say the words, *My sexual needs are important,* over and over in your mind. Believe them!

You don't have to take time to unwind *every* day (although that's the ideal, of course). But you do need to make this a part of your weekly routine. And if it's only once a week or once every two weeks that you can relax enough to enjoy a sensual moment with your partner or yourself, then that's fine. Just as long as when you do so, it's with a positive attitude and the desire to do something special for *yourself.*

If this doesn't meet your partner's needs, you may have to mention that it's quality, not quantity, you're after. Remind him or her that masturbation is a great option when one person wants sex more often than the other.

And when you do start to be sexual (whether with a partner or on your own), there is one more thing you can do. Try taking a little more time than you have in the past (at least an extra twenty minutes) to fantasize, cuddle, talk, and caress *before* moving to sexual activity. This will give you a chance to consciously switch *off* from the busy day and on to your sensual and personal needs.

**A word of warning:** it's very easy to start making changes this way and then forget to keep them up. It only takes one or two days of losing sight of that thought, *My sexual needs are important,* and— quick as a flash—you'll be back into your old habits.

Here are some suggestions to keep you focused on making changes:

- If it helps, leave signs around the house which say, MY SEXUAL FEELINGS ARE A PRIORITY, TOO. Tuck them into drawers, wardrobes, or other places you go to frequently (the fridge?).
- Remind yourself of how it was when you were less busy, gave sex more importance and had fewer responsibilities.
- Picture in detail a nice sexual memory. Remember how it actually *felt.* If you have no nice memories, then daydream about how a nice sexual moment would look and feel. It's so easy to push these memories and dreams to one side and think that sex is not worth the effort.
- Most importantly, work on that attitude of yours—the one that says being busy is the only way to like yourself or to be successful.
- Just remember why you started reading this book—and why you have kept on reading.

You may find doing the Personal and Couple Change Programs a good way to keep you focused on this new approach. To start with, the Programs require you to set aside time for exercises that are aimed at helping you to feel relaxed, sensuous, and sexy. Learning how to fit the Programs into your busy day will be an important step towards having orgasms.

# life became full of stress and upset |

THERE ARE THREE kinds of women who find that feelings of stress and upset affect their ability to have an orgasm. The *first* type are those who have a stressful event (or events) in their lives and are simply reacting—as anyone would. The situation leaves them worried about what to do or what's going to happen in the future. Naturally, these emotions will interfere with sexual arousal. How can you relax and get lost in the sexual moment when your mind is on other worrying matters?

If this describes you, give some thought to whether your life is going to return to "normal" in the near future. If so, perhaps you shouldn't worry too much about not feeling orgasms, and (if you have a partner) concentrate instead on having some close times, so that you feel supported. Talk to him or her about it and see if you can agree that, for the moment, it will be enough to spend some time cuddling, doing gentle massaging or going to the movies, and so on. You might feel aroused on some occasions, but not on others. Don't pressure yourself about this. Simply accept that this is the way you are for the moment. In other words, give yourself permission to *not* have orgasms at this time.

On the other hand, if you follow the suggestions I gave above to women who are too busy, you may find that making a special effort to get into a relaxed mood is just what you need to distract yourself from the stress around you. Try it. You may be surprised to find that switching off from your worries for a short while can give you more energy to keep going (and a brief time to enjoy sexual arousal again).

The *second* type of woman who finds that feelings of stress and upset affect her ability to have an orgasm is one who worries about most things. She's often anxious and uptight about little things that aren't going right in her life. Actually, she's quite a worrier.

---

I suppose I've always been a worrier, just like my father. But I used to get by without it affecting my sexual feelings. What's changed?

---

It could be anything. I hate to say it but, as we get older, some of us seem to cope less effectively with stress. I don't know whether it's just the effect of aging, or whether getting older brings with it so much more responsibility. I suspect it's both.

What this means, dear reader, is that if you're the worrying type, and you want to orgasm again, you'll need to find another way of dealing with the world. Being a worrier often means "expecting the worst," focusing on things that *could* go wrong. This, as you know, makes it hard to relax and enjoy yourself in most situations, *including* sex.

I suggest you see a psychologist, who can help you to understand why you're a worrier and how you can change it.

You might also consider doing the Personal and Couple Change Programs. They'll encourage you to relax and focus on something positive: your sexuality.

The *third* type of woman who is aware that stress and upset affect her ability to have an orgasm is the person who finds it hard to let go of the grief or deep sadness she feels inside. There are many possible reasons for this. I've seen women who, years after the death of a loved one, were still grieving as if it had happened yesterday. Some believe that to stop feeling it this much would be a sign they didn't care any more. Others, unable to cry fully at the time of the death, have never finished grieving.

&#8450;

REGARDLESS OF WHY you're stressed and upset, let me remind you that bottling up your feelings is bad for your health, peace of mind, and sexuality. If possible, find someone to open up to. It doesn't matter who it is—a friend, the stranger sitting on the bus next to you, a therapist, your partner. . . .

Research shows us that women who get support from others are able to cope with stressful events better than those who try to do things alone. If you're too shy or independent to speak to someone, you might have to settle for whispering into your cat's/dog's ear. Better still, get some professional help, so that you can learn to talk to someone without fear of being a burden or a failure.

By the way, you may need to put sex on hold while you work through your emotions. However, a cuddle or massage may be just what you need. Don't worry if this makes you want to cry. It's a perfectly natural reaction for many women.

Remember to tell your partner if you need to stop being sexual at the moment. Explain that you can't have high levels of sadness *and* sexual pleasure at the same time.

# life became boring

BOREDOM OFTEN SNEAKS up on us when we're least expecting it. It seems to happen without any effort on our part. However, just admitting to being bored has probably started you on the road to change. It's hard to recognize that life is dull without feeling restless and looking for a way out of it.

The first step to overcoming boredom is to allow yourself to dream about things being different. I often get bored people to write a list of what would give them a *buzz* or a *feeling of excitement*. Try this yourself:

## What would give me a buzz
*right now!*

1. _____

2. _____

3. _____

4. _____

Now, place a check next to those items on your list which can be carried out at this time in your life. Is there anything stopping you from following them through? If so, can these obstacles be overcome?

Answering these questions should give you an idea of what needs to be done to get rid of the boredom. If there seem to be too many obstacles or you're not sure what's stopping you from making the necessary changes, a session or two with a psychologist or well-trained counselor should help.

What if your boredom is solely in connection with your sexual activity? Let's say you aren't bored with life in general, but the predictability of your sex life is driving you crazy. And this makes it impossible to really get turned on.

How can you get "lost in the sexual moment" if you already know exactly what that sexual moment is going to be? How can you feel passionate when sex is predictable and unadventurous? The answer is, you can't, because there's no excitement to trigger your sexual feelings.

There's only one thing to do: make your lovemaking *less* predictable and *more* adventurous. If you have a partner, that means talking about the problem with him or her.

---

But I'm worried my partner will see this as an attack on our relationship. She's really sensitive to criticism. What if it starts an argument and makes sex worse than it is?

---

Well, you're certainly painting a pretty gloomy picture, but I realize our attempts to improve things can sometimes create further problems. You may have to think carefully about how you communicate with your partner. Try to word your comments in a way that doesn't put blame on either of you.

If you use words that seem to be an attack *(I'm not happy with the way you make love)*, then you'll get a defensive response *(Well, it's all your fault, you never seem interested)*. If you try starting with how you feel about the situation, you might do better.

---

What about something like, "Honey, I know I'm drifting off when we make love. I don't like it any more than you do. Maybe it would help if we tried doing things a bit differently . . . you know . . . have a bit more fun, spark things up. I'm sure it would help me. What do you think?"

---

Yes, that sounds great. Unless your relationship is in serious trouble, a chat along these lines should start the ball rolling. You may even find that your partner is also bored and has been trying to figure out how to tell *you*.

I would also *strongly* suggest the two of you do the Couple Change Program. It usually helps to get people out of a sexual rut.

Read chapter 14 first, and then give it to your partner to read. If you both feel ready to do it, don't waste any time. Start this week.

If your partner isn't interested, then you'd better start talking even more directly about your boredom. Otherwise, your difficulties could turn into a relationship issue rather than a sexual one.

If you don't have a regular partner, but rather different partners from time to time, you may not feel it's appropriate to talk about your boredom with them. Of course, you still need to figure out why you get bored, especially if it happens with most of your partners.

For example, do you choose partners who aren't interested in being sexual in the way you like to be? If so, why do you keep selecting people who always disappoint you? Then again, perhaps you stop yourself from letting go. You may feel shy or awkward about being more adventurous. Try to understand why. If necessary, talk to a therapist about becoming more open with your sexual passion.

Finally, what if your boredom with sexual activity occurs when you're touching yourself? I think you probably know what to do by now: you can vary the way you do it, the parts of your body you touch, where you are during masturbation, the fantasies you have, and even when you masturbate.

Some women get into a routine of masturbating in the same way and at the same time and with the same fantasy. They're not masturbating in a way that's fun, simply doing what they always do. Break the habit. It can be fun trying.

## too little time to get highly aroused |

THERE IS A simple and a not-so-simple answer to this cause of your orgasm difficulties. The easy part is that all you need to do is take more time for relaxing and touching before trying to build your sexual arousal to orgasm levels. The hard part may be finding or making the time.

Try to allow *at least* twenty minutes of caressing, stroking, and cuddling in your lovemaking before you even think about building your arousal and having an orgasm. This will give you time to relax, unwind from the day and switch your mind from being a mother, partner, manager (or whatever role you've been in for the previous hour or two) to being *a lover.* You can't get highly aroused if your mind is still at work or changing diapers.

You may need longer than twenty minutes. Experiment with different lengths of time to find out what works best for you. And listen to what your body is telling you. Is it tense? Then take more time. Listen to your mind. Is it racing with ideas? Are you having trouble putting your attention on what is happening *now*? Then you need more time to get into a sexual mood.

And don't forget to tell your partner how you're feeling. He or she isn't a mind reader, no matter how much love they feel for you.

---

Shouldn't my partner be able to sense what I'm
feeling? After all, we've been together four years.

---

After four years your partner is probably quite good at figuring out whether or not you're relaxed and getting aroused. But *you* are the only person who can read your body cues accurately. And if your partner is beginning to get turned on sexually, he or she may mistakenly think the two of you have similar levels of sexual arousal. Remember, it's not easy gauging a partner's feelings if you're caught up in your own sexual pleasure.

By the way, giving yourself extra time can work just as well if you're on your own and pleasuring yourself.

---

But how do I make this extra time?
There's so much to do each day.

---

I suggest you read the previous section in this chapter on "being a busy person." *Firstly,* you will need to believe that taking the time to enjoy sex (and have orgasms) is important. If you see everything else as more important, you'll *never* take time for sexual pleasure. *Secondly,* you'll need to decide which *non*sexual activity will have to wait. This doesn't have to occur every day or even every week. But *sometimes* you need to give more importance to your sexual needs. Remember, I'm only suggesting a minimum of twenty minutes.

# 9

# changing your
# personal style

I N THIS CHAPTER I'll help you to change the way your own attitudes, emotions and behaviors interfere with sexual arousal. Your job, dear reader, is to look at what you do *without* judging or blaming yourself (which I know many women do). Nothing will change if you can't show yourself a bit of kindness and caring.

## being goal-focused

BEING GOAL-FOCUSED usually means being *future-*focused, always thinking ahead. Of course, most of us do have to think ahead at different times. We might be planning a birthday celebration, worrying about a job interview next week, saving money for a holiday, and so on.

However, some people spend *most* of their time thinking about the future. They pay little attention to the present and often miss a lot of

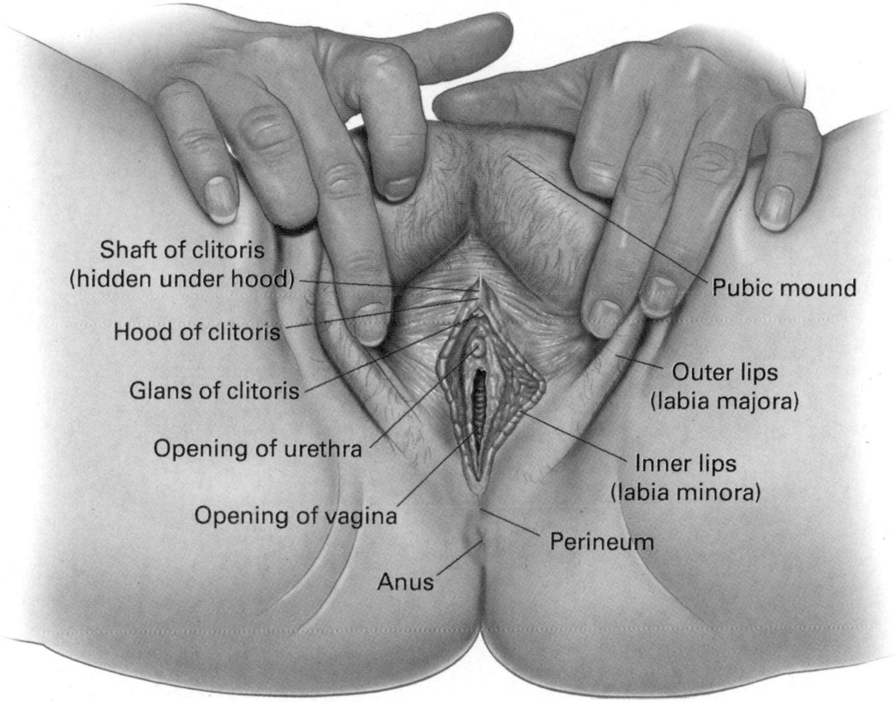

Shaft of clitoris
(hidden under hood)

Hood of clitoris

Glans of clitoris

Opening of urethra

Opening of vagina

Anus

Pubic mound

Outer lips
(labia majora)

Inner lips
(labia minora)

Perineum

**Figure 1**

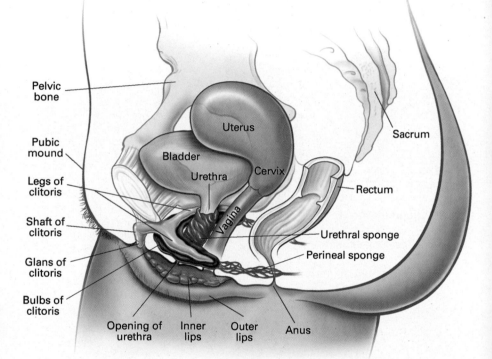

Pelvic bone

Pubic mound

Legs of clitoris

Shaft of clitoris

Glans of clitoris

Bulbs of clitoris

Uterus

Bladder

Urethra

Cervix

Vagina

Sacrum

Rectum

Urethral sponge

Perineal sponge

Opening of urethra

Inner lips

Outer lips

Anus

**Figure 2**

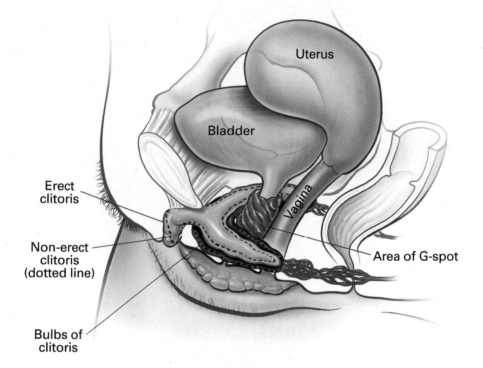

Uterus

Bladder

Erect
clitoris

Non-erect
clitoris
(dotted line)

Vagina

Area of G-spot

Bulbs of
clitoris

**Figure 3**

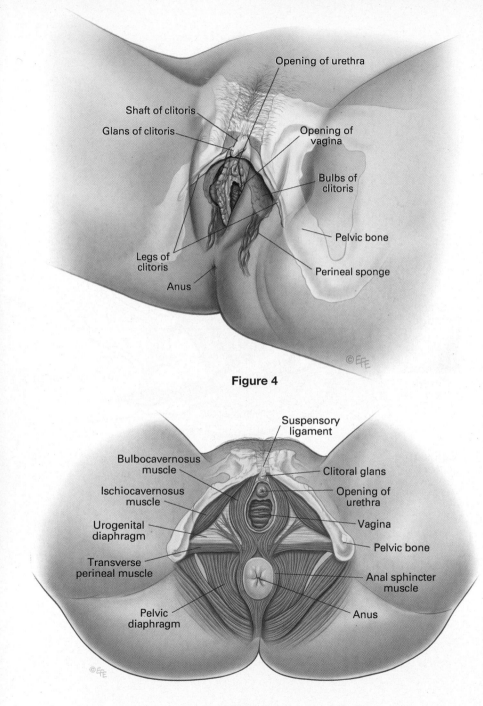

**Figure 4**

**Figure 5**

what is going on around them. In their minds they have *things-that-HAVE-to-be-done.*

They're very good at concentrating on these goals. What they're *not* good at, though, is noticing how they're being affected by those around them and what they're feeling (emotionally and physically). They may also have trouble enjoying simple pleasures such as watching a sunset or listening to the birds sing. They find it hard to just be. They always have to be *doing.*

In a sexual situation, women like this often have difficulty getting aroused. Can you see why? Being sexual requires you to be aware of what's happening right now and to enjoy the present moment. In a sexual situation, that means:

- being aware of what emotions you feel
- noticing the sensations in your body
- having your attention on what you're doing
- having your attention on what your partner is doing
- being aware of, but not *thinking* about (for example, planning or worrying about) what's going on
- not judging what's going on

And most importantly,

- not setting orgasm as the *goal* to strive for.

---

Whoa, I'll have to make a few changes to be able to do what you're suggesting. I don't notice what's going on OUTSIDE the bedroom, let alone IN it.

---

That's true for many goal-focused people. It's a personal style, usually learned from a parent who did (maybe still does) the same thing. But it *is* possible to change and become more aware of the present. Let's start with trying to change your style "outside the bedroom," as you put it.

I find the following exercise very helpful:

> For the next three days,
> ask yourself every hour
> (where possible, of course),
>
> **What am I feeling right now?**

Don't worry if you can't answer your own question at first. When you're not used to noticing your feelings or body reactions, it can be difficult to "read" what is there. Keep doing the exercise, however, and eventually you'll start noticing more about yourself.

Some women find it difficult to put into words what they're feeling. If this is also a problem for you, learn to identify your emotions by first noticing where you feel tense or relaxed in your body. For example, you might become aware that you feel tense in the stomach area. So notice, *I'm tight in the stomach*—even if you don't understand what this is about.

Eventually you'll come to understand what the sensation of tightness is telling you. You might become aware that it seems linked to *worry* about a child who is sick or to *panic* about a work deadline that you're battling to meet, or to some other problem.

The reason I want you to do the exercise every hour for those first three days is that it helps to break the habit of concentrating only on the next task (goal) you've planned (the future), while ignoring yourself in the present.

After three days, you should spend another week asking the same question, *What am I feeling right now?* three times a day. I suggest once in the morning, once during the day and once at night, to make it easier to remember.

By practicing this exercise you can teach yourself to focus on the present. You'll also feel the difference between being in the present and being in the future. Don't be surprised if you start to feel less exhausted. It's more tiring always running after the future than it is taking notice of the present.

NOW, IT'S NOT enough to simply learn how to be aware of yourself in the present. You also have to learn how to enjoy the present, *without having to give it some purpose.*

Do you find this difficult? To find out, turn to the next page and answer the questions in the box.

## enjoying the present quiz

1. Can you take a nice leisurely stroll (without having to walk fast in order to feel that what you're doing is something "useful" —such as getting you fit)?     Yes ☐    No ☐

2. Do you enjoy moments of watching a sunset or waves rolling in on a beach or the wind in the trees (without getting impatient at the time you're wasting and moving on after a few moments)?     Yes ☐    No ☐

3. Are you able to take a bath, listen to some music, or read a book (without getting restless and needing to do something else)?     Yes ☐    No ☐

If you answered no to any of these questions, you're like many goal-focused women who find it difficult to indulge in leisure or pleasure time where there is "no useful purpose" other than to relax and enjoy themselves.

The problem arises, of course, when you place sex in the "no-useful-purpose" category (yes, there are many women who do this!). Can you see the difficulty you have? After a short time you'll get impatient and want to move onto some other activity. You might even pretend to have an orgasm just to get sex over and done with as quickly as possible.

**In other words, you won't hang around long enough to reach orgasm.**

So let me suggest something that will help you change your style of doing things. I have another exercise for you.

---

Choose three leisure activities that you've never done in a truly relaxed way, or never done at all because they required too much relaxation time.

Make a definite date with yourself to try each one. Your "goal" should be simply to enjoy yourself and be focused on the present.

---

For example, try taking a bath while sipping some wine, reading a book, or just staring into space. Go for a slow walk with your only purpose being to relax, notice your surroundings and enjoy yourself. Go somewhere where you can watch a sunset. And try to enjoy it. Notice the colors, the smells around you, how you feel, and so on. It doesn't matter what you do, as long as you're learning to be present-focused.

Recognize that enjoying yourself in a relaxed way and taking time to notice what's going on around you is important for *your* well-being.

THE SAME EXERCISES can be used in the sexual area.

If you're expressing yourself sexually, either on your own or with a partner, ask the same question, *What am I feeling right now?* Again, don't worry if you're stumped for words. The important thing is to ask the question, because this teaches you to focus on the present. You'll never get an answer if you don't remember to ask the question.

Many women find that becoming tuned into the present moment makes them more aware of the exact moment when they switch off their sexual feelings. They also learn why that happens. It's common, for example, to discover that the change in sexual arousal is linked to shifting thoughts from the present to something to be done later that day, tomorrow or next week (the future).

The next time you're involved in sexual activity, allow yourself to take time to relax and enjoy it. If you become impatient, try saying, *It's good for me to simply enjoy what's happening.* Say this as many times as you like, because it will help to stop the other thought at the back of your mind. You know the one I mean: *This isn't getting me anywhere, I might as well get up and do* _____ (fill in whichever task fits).

I would also strongly recommend you do the Personal Change Program. It will give you a chance to learn to focus on yourself and your sexual feelings, without being distracted by another person.

Later, if appropriate, you should follow up with the Couple Change Program. This will allow you to take what you've learned from the Personal Program and use it to become more present-focused with your partner.

℘

ONE FINAL POINT about women who are goal-focused. If you're also a perfectionist, you're likely to see the lack of orgasm as a personal failure. I'm sure I don't need to tell you how much damage this belief can do. What can you do about this? Let's start with the idea that there are good and bad parts to perfectionism.

The good side is that it makes us always try very hard to do our best. As a result, we may do something better than someone who isn't a perfectionist. Some jobs need close attention to detail, and that's where perfectionists come into their own.

The bad side of perfectionism is that, apart from driving our non-perfectionist partners absolutely crazy, it means living constantly with the anxiety of not meeting the very high standards we set for ourselves. We don't know how to relax and do things in a less perfect way.

So, you don't have to go through a total personality change: you can hold onto the good side of perfectionism and try to reduce the bad side. You may find working with a psychologist helpful with this. Understanding why we've learned to be perfectionists can be very interesting.

Now, let's come back to you and your orgasm difficulty. Many perfectionists will switch off sexually rather than risk failure. In addition, there are the "turn-off thoughts" to deal with. Have you noticed negative thoughts that pop into your head? Do any of the following examples seem familiar?

- *I'm a complete failure.*
- *I'm useless at sex.*
- *It's no use trying because I never get there.*
- *I should be able to orgasm like other women.*
- *If I can't have an orgasm every time, I'm a failure.*

By now, you know that thoughts such as these will send your arousal down into the deepest valley. Your first step to change, then, is learning how to be less focused on the need to be perfect in everything. You also need to know how to change the negative thoughts into positive ones. You may want to work with a therapist on this.

I'd also suggest you do the Personal Change Program exactly as I describe it. *Don't* try to do it faster or skip steps because you think this is a better way to go. It's not! Try to relax and accept that you are just like everyone else and must give yourself time to learn new skills (and unlearn old ones).

## needing to stay in control of emotions |

IF YOU'VE IDENTIFIED that you like to stay in control of your emotions, the next step is to try to understand why. Look at the *Why I Control My Emotions Quiz* on the next page. Write down your answers to the questions.

# why I control my emotions quiz

1. Are you simply following the ways of your parents, who also held back emotionally?

   Yes ☐  No ☐

2. Are you *uncomfortable* or *afraid* when you feel strong emotions?

   Yes ☐  No ☐

   *If you answered yes, why is this?*

   Are you scared you'll be totally overwhelmed by them?

   Yes ☐  No ☐

   Are you nervous about embarrassing yourself?

   Yes ☐  No ☐

3. Are you someone who is naturally reserved and private and sees letting go of emotions as being too exposing?

   Yes ☐  No ☐

4. Do you feel *guilty* about enjoying yourself too much?

   Yes ☐  No ☐

5. Are there any emotions you feel comfortable expressing (e.g., anger)?

   Yes ☐  No ☐

   What are these? _____

6. Is it easy for you to feel pleasant emotions, like fun, joy, happiness, humor and so on?

   Yes ☐  No ☐

7. Are you a person who likes to do everything in a rational way?

   Yes ☐  No ☐

8. Do you find emotions "messy"?

   Yes ☐  No ☐

Take some time to think about these questions. After writing down your answers, find out what they tell you about the way you *think of* and *deal with* emotions.

Next, see if you can identify what you'd like to change in the way you handle emotions. Write these in the space below:

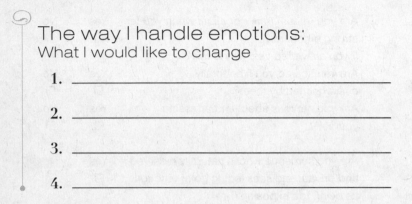

## The way I handle emotions:
### What I would like to change

1. _____

2. _____

3. _____

4. _____

Check that you're not confusing what you'd *like* to change with what you feel you *should* change. There's a big difference between the two. Wanting to change will motivate you to try things differently. Believing you *have* to change will make you half-hearted in your attempts, and it's unlikely that anything will happen.

Think about what you need to do to make these changes. Just being aware of the problem areas might be enough to start behaving differently. You may also find talking to a psychologist or a well-trained counselor helpful.

It doesn't matter how you do it. Just remember, learning to be less controlled emotionally is going to be important in helping you to be more aroused sexually. So give some time to learning how to open up.

IF YOU HAVE no problems handling emotions in general, but find *sexual* emotions difficult, try the next exercise.

I'm now going to ask you to imagine a sexual scene. First read the description of the scene on the next page, then shut your eyes and try and imagine it in as much detail as you can. *Be aware of how you're feeling and reacting as you do this.* After you have imagined the scene for about three minutes, open your eyes and continue reading.

---

## the scene

*Imagine you're in a sexual situation that you find very pleasant. The scene excites you sexually, and you begin to get turned on. Your sexual feelings are like warm syrup flowing through your body, and you feel yourself being swept along with the flow.*

*Gradually you become more aroused. You feel very excited and become more and more turned on. You feel yourself moving with desire and hear your sounds of passion. At this moment there is no other world—just you and your sexual pleasure.*

---

*Imagine this scene before reading beyond this point.*

Notice how you're feeling at this moment. Shut your eyes so you can focus on your body. Identify where you're feeling relaxed and where you're tense. What do these reactions tell you?

STOP and do this now.

---

Wow, I actually feel tense. It began when I imagined really letting myself go sexually. I felt my stomach tighten up, and I couldn't breathe properly.

---

Yes, even an imaginary exercise can have this effect. Sounds like the thought of letting go sexually makes you anxious or frightened, doesn't it? Stop and think about what your reactions might mean.

There may be others who felt enjoyment doing the exercise. This would suggest a different kind of problem with sexual passion. I want to talk about each of these reactions, beginning with feeling anxious and afraid.

Why do you feel afraid of your sexual passion? There can be many reasons. *Sexual fears* are usually formed in three ways:

- By a real situation, happening in your life *at this moment*, which makes it impossible for you to become more than a little aroused. For example, a sexual partner who frequently criticizes you or threatens you.
- By past sexual events that still affect you in a negative way, even though you know there's nothing to be afraid of now. Let me give you some examples:
  - You were frightened in childhood or adolescence by seeing someone highly aroused and *now you become anxious at the sight of someone really turned on.*
  - You walked in on someone having sex (for example, a brother, your parents, a cousin), were embarrassed, but found it stimulating at the same time, *and now you become uncomfortable when you get "too" sexually aroused.*
  - You felt afraid when you were being sexually abused, *and now you get frightened when your partner gets aroused, even though you know it's a loving relationship.*
  - As a teenager you became sexually aroused during petting and felt scared that you might go further and get pregnant, *and now you become tense whenever your arousal gets beyond a certain level.*
  - You were once criticized when you were expressing sexual passion, *and now you feel on edge waiting for a rejection from your partner—even though you know this isn't going to happen.*
- By negative and wrong teaching about sexuality: for example, being told that women look ugly during orgasm, or that sex will hurt.

These experiences can teach us to be afraid of our own sexual arousal. Take a few moments to think about your situation, and see if you can find what it is you're afraid of *now.* Don't worry if it doesn't seem very rational. Try to look for answers that really do appear to explain your reactions, not ones you believe *should* explain them. Check whether your fears are triggered by something in the present or the past.

If there's something or someone in your life *right now* making it hard for you to show sexual passion

**. . . changing *you* may not be the answer.**

Instead, you'll need to change your situation. If this can't be done, the only alternative is to accept the circumstances as they are and take the pressure off yourself to have orgasms.

If your fears seem to come from past events *that can't be changed,* and there's no logical reason for you to still feel this way, you'll have to take a different approach.

**What needs to be changed is the way you link the past with the present.**

The first step is to find ways of reminding yourself that *the past is different from the present.* The positive statements in the next box can help you to do this.

---

## positive statements
### to cancel fears of sexual passion

- There's no need to be afraid anymore; I'm with _____ (partner's name) and I'm safe.
- I'm an adult and it's now okay for me to let go sexually.
- The situation/person that frightened me into controlling my sexual feelings in the past can no longer affect me. It's okay to enjoy my sexual feelings the way I want.
- Now that I'm an adult, I can choose to be sexual the way I want. I don't have to let the past control me.

---

Choose the phrases that seem to fit you best, and say them *out loud* right now. Do this several times.

The next time you're in a sexual situation and feel yourself switching off, say the phrases to yourself, listening carefully to the words. In time you should find yourself relaxing and less anxious about feeling the strength of your sexual pleasure. You will then be able to build your arousal to levels high enough for you to orgasm.

You may find it helpful to do the Personal Change Program. This is a nice gentle way to learn how to let your sexual arousal build more strongly. If you have a partner, you may want to continue with the Couple Change Program so that you can learn to express your sexual passion in front of another person.

However, if thinking about the past continues to bring up emotions such as fear, anxiety or panic, you're probably not yet ready to make changes in the sexual area. Get some help from a psychologist or therapist who can show you how to work through these feelings. You may never forget the events that sparked your fears. That's understandable. But you can get to a point where what happened no longer has the ability to prevent you from having an orgasm.

Now, let me talk to those of you who *didn't* feel anxious or fearful as you imagined the sexual scene in the exercise I gave earlier. What could explain your positive reaction to the exercise?

Firstly, you may be feeling *ready* to let yourself go sexually, but don't know how to put it into practice, especially with someone else present.

---

Well, I don't want to scare anyone off.
They might think I'm a nympho or something!

---

A quick translation for other readers. Nympho is shorthand for nymphomaniac, a DREADFUL, DREADFUL word that describes a woman who is *too* sexual *(whatever that means!)*. This word should be banned. Is there a similar word for men? Of course not! Being *highly* sexual is seen as normal in men. But when women act in the same way, they're called *too* sexual.

Why the difference? Probably because the people who invented the word *nymphomaniac* considered it wrong for women to experience the freedom, strength, and equality that comes from fully enjoying sexual passion. It's a very interesting example of how society has contributed to making women feel bad about their sexual feelings. Don't let me get started on that one.

The easiest way of learning how to let go of the control over your sexual feelings is to practice—on your own. If you already masturbate, try touching yourself to the point where you usually switch off. Remind yourself that you now feel ready to let go. Look forward to your feelings growing stronger. Relax and continue touching yourself. If you become uncomfortable with the intensity of your feelings, take a break and focus on thinking positively. When ready, continue touching. You might want to do the Personal Change Program, perhaps skipping over the first two steps.

If you don't yet masturbate, begin with the Personal Change Program. It will slowly lead you into feeling stronger and more intense sexual feelings without fear. If you're in a relationship, you may also find it useful to follow the Couple Change Program.

# difficulty showing sexual passion |

SOME WOMEN CAN fully enjoy their sexual passion on their own, but find it difficult to do so with a partner. During sex we reveal a side of ourselves that isn't seen in everyday life. To do this comfortably with a partner, we need to feel secure and relaxed enough to show our sexual self to others. This means showing:

- how you look when you're aroused
- the noises you make when aroused
- how you move your body when aroused
- what you like done to you to become aroused
- how vulnerable you become when aroused
- how romantic you are when aroused
- how different (wild?) you are when aroused
- how much you enjoy sex

Some women find it embarrassing to be this open with any sexual partner. Others are awkward at *some* times, or with *some* partners, and not others.

To get highly aroused and to orgasm, it's important that you're at ease with letting your sexual passion be seen by a partner. If not, you'll probably get halfway up the arousal hill and then freeze with embarrassment.

> It's funny, but I do feel very awkward about opening up sexually with my partner. In the twenty years we've been together, he thinks I'm this nice conservative woman, not a passionate one. But I had no problems a year ago when I had an affair. Is that weird?

No, it's quite common for women to feel relaxed about showing their sexual passion to one kind of person (for example, a new lover) but not to another kind (for example, a regular partner who hasn't seen them that way). Being with a new lover can make it easier to show sexual passion because there are no expectations of how you should be— as there would be with a partner who's known you for twenty years!

So, your difficulty with showing sexual passion may simply be a difficulty being yourself.

Women find it difficult to show passion to another person for other reasons. Sometimes a negative experience has taught them to hold back (for example, someone laughing at the way you expressed yourself sexually).

Sometimes we imagine something terrible happening if we let ourselves go sexually in front of someone else. These fears are often imaginary.

Try the next exercise to learn more about yourself:

## what do i imagine will happen?
### finish the sentence below:

If I show my sexual passion, I'm worried the following will happen:

1. _____

2. _____

3. _____

4. _____

*Write down the things you imagine will happen.*

Now you have something to work on. If your worries are realistic, it may be perfectly natural for you to be unable to let go enough to orgasm. For example, if your partner gets embarrassed by the sounds of you enjoying your sexual pleasure, you may be so busy controlling yourself that you lose your arousal.

In this case, you need to try to change the situation so you can be yourself. You could talk to your partner about the effect his or her embarrassment is having on you. You could see a therapist to help your partner become less awkward and controlled. And so on.

However, if you can see that your concerns or fears are more imaginary than real, then you'll find it helpful to remind yourself of this during sex with a partner. Tell yourself there's no *real* reason for not showing your sexual passion.

If you can, talk to your partner. You may be surprised with his or her reaction. I once counseled a woman who controlled her sexual passion during oral sex because she was embarrassed at ejaculating when she became highly aroused. She could happily show sexual passion in all other ways except oral sex. Eventually she talked with her partner about this and was amazed to find that he saw this as a turn-on, not a turn-off, as she'd feared.

So, if possible, share your fears. Let your partner know you're having difficulty being open about your feelings. During sex, try using humor and fun to lighten the atmosphere. Be patient. It may take a little time for you to break down the barriers.

And, most importantly, accept that your sexual passion is part of you, and needs to be expressed, just as do other parts of you.

If you'd like more guidance in making changes with your partner, the Couple Change Program could be just what you need.

# feeling guilt |

FEELING GUILTY DURING sex is a sure sign you've learned a nasty little message about it being wrong to express or enjoy sexual feelings—*your* sexual feelings, to be exact. If this is the case, feeling aroused will probably make you think you've done something "wrong" and that it's your "fault." You may not know what it is that you've done. But this doesn't matter. You'll feel "guilty" anyway.

Not surprisingly, *guilt* and *orgasms* don't go together too well. So, if you want to learn how to let your sexual feelings build to orgasm, it means letting go of the guilt.

### To orgasm,

- We need to be able to focus on our own arousal, body sensations, and feelings *without guilt* (or, for that matter, fear, embarrassment, or shame).
- We need to feel that it's acceptable to enjoy ourselves.
- We need to stop worrying about everyone else's needs and give more attention to our own.

**And we need to do this without thinking we're selfish**.

Don't be worried if you have trouble accepting this message. Many, *many* women have the same problem. As girls, we've been encouraged to be obedient, conform to our parents' wishes, and focus on caring for others rather than ourselves.

No wonder that, as adults, we find it hard to recognize *our* needs and wishes as important. No wonder that we find it hard to put aside daily responsibilities and focus on sex and having fun.

---

But if I think only of
my sexual needs,
that IS selfish.
What about other people
who rely on me to
be there for them?

---

Wait . . . I didn't say anything about giving up entirely on your responsibilities. But what sort of life is it if you always focus on the needs of others? What sort of life do you have if you never feel right about enjoying yourself? You *do* want to have some fun, don't you?

> I suppose I do, but I never feel right when I'm
> having a good time and know someone else wants
> me to do something for them. I feel I have to do
> what they want first.

Well, maybe that's where your orgasm problems start. Thinking these kinds of thoughts—*especially* during sex—will take your attention away from enjoying yourself. This, in turn, will stop your arousal from building to orgasm. The question is, are you prepared to care for yourself as much as you care for others?

And are you prepared to give up your guilt? Funnily enough, some women feel comforted by their guilt. It makes them feel they're a "good" person. So, they're half-hearted about making changes. If this picture fits you, *and you feel frustrated by your resistance to change*, see a professional therapist who can help you to understand what keeps you stuck in the guilt.

If you feel ready to let the guilt go, it will mean changing some beliefs. For example, the belief that if you're enjoying yourself, it means you're a "bad," lazy, or selfish person. Or the belief that it's wrong to feel sexual pleasure.

Take some time to reflect about how you came to think this way. Be aware of how you feel as you recall childhood experiences that taught you to feel guilty. Ask yourself whether the guilt you feel *now* about enjoying yourself is simply a habit, something you've been taught to do.

When you feel ready to learn how to enjoy yourself without guilt, try the next exercise. In the box below are some positive (antiguilt) statements.

## getting over guilt
### about enjoying myself

- It's time for me to enjoy life.
- I was taught to feel guilty about having fun—I don't have to feel this way any more.
- It's okay to take time from my responsibilities to enjoy myself.

- I want to decide whether I'll relax and have some fun. I don't want my childhood to decide for me.
- It's natural to take time to enjoy myself. I don't have to feel guilty about this any longer.

*Write in any others you think of :*

- _____

- _____

Read through each one *out loud* (it's not the same if you say them in your head). Do this several times. Notice how you feel as you say them.

Now, for one week, say these statements to yourself *twice a day*. Don't forget even one day. And keep saying them, even if, at first, the words sound strange. It won't be long before they feel *right*.

The next step is learning to put your new way of thinking into practice. Try taking a half hour once or twice a week to do something enjoyable, something you previously felt guilty about doing. Keep doing this until you feel completely comfortable and relaxed. If you feel even a twinge of guilt, say your antiguilt statements immediately.

&copy;

NOW, LET'S TURN to learning to enjoy yourself *sexually* without guilt. The same three steps can be used here. Firstly, take some time to try to understand where you learned to think and feel guilty about sexual pleasure. Be aware of how you feel. Recognize that these early lessons don't have to apply to you as an adult. Admit that these childhood lessons taught you the *wrong* thing about sexual pleasure.

Secondly, start thinking positively. I've made a few suggestions below, but you can add any others that come to mind. Read through each positive thought out loud. Notice how you feel as you say them.

# getting over guilt
## about enjoying sexual pleasure

- It's time for me to enjoy life—and that includes my sexual feelings.
- I was taught to feel guilty about feeling sexy. I don't have to feel this way any more.
- It's okay to take time from my responsibilities to enjoy my sexual feelings.
- I want to decide whether I'll have an orgasm. I don't want my childhood experiences to decide for me.
- Being sexually turned on is natural. I don't have to feel guilty about this any longer.

*Write in any others you think of :*

- _____

- _____

Just as before, for one week say these statements to yourself *twice a day*. Keep saying them until you feel comfortable with each thought. You're now ready to use them during sex. Before you begin any sexual activity, say them to yourself. If, during sex, you get a twinge of guilt, say them again. Don't worry if it takes a little while for the guilt to disappear. It can take time to undo the negative effects of guilt. Keep practicing and let the changes take place at their own pace.

If you have any difficulties with these suggestions, see a psychologist or experienced therapist, who can help you to understand why.

## trying too hard to please a partner

DO YOU STOP yourself from becoming highly aroused by trying too hard to please your partner? If so, there are some quite simple changes you can make. Let's begin by looking at your approach to life and sex.

Some women try too hard to please *everyone*. They may believe this is the best way to express caring of others. Or they may feel guilty if they think about themselves. Perhaps they're driven by a belief of not being good enough and are trying to prove they're a nice person.

Being *this* caring of others can be a wonderful quality, provided you don't ignore *your* needs. Otherwise, you may become resentful because nobody seems to pay attention to what makes *you* happy (even though you act as if your needs aren't important).

If you want to stop this resentment from affecting your relationships with others, you must keep a balance between meeting other people's needs *and* your own needs. But to do this, you need to hold a positive attitude towards yourself. You have to believe that *you* are worthwhile. If you're not sure whether you feel positive about yourself, try the next exercise.

---

Say the following sentences out loud,

**My needs are important, too.**
**It's okay if I also pay attention to what I need**
**to make me happy.**

---

Shut your eyes and say this twice more, and listen carefully to what you're saying. Does it feel *right* to say this? As you say this sentence, do you feel strong, pleased, determined? If so, the next step is to make this message work in the sexual setting.

If, however, you feel uneasy when talking about your needs, it probably means the idea that you must please everyone *first* is a very strongly held belief. Trying to change strong beliefs can make us feel guilty, disloyal and uncomfortable.

Now, I don't want to tell you to give up this belief. But do understand that this belief will follow you into the bedroom. You simply won't get highly aroused if your only concern is with your partner's sexual satisfaction. So, hang on to your belief if you wish, but realize that you may have to live with your orgasm difficulties.

However, I suggest you try the Couple Change Program before

making up your mind on this matter. It may help you to become more comfortable with expressing *your* sexual needs. You may also find it useful to see a psychologist and get a better understanding of why it's so difficult for you to look after your needs.

For those of you who feel ready to change the belief, here are a few tips on how to get there:

- Be prepared to give your own sexual needs just as much importance during lovemaking as you give your partner's.
- Learn to shift your attention back and forth between your partner and yourself (without guilt). At first you'll have to make a special effort to be more aware of how you're reacting physically and emotionally. Try not to analyse what's happening, otherwise you'll start thinking too much and your arousal will most certainly disappear. Just notice. Eventually it will become easier to pay attention to yourself without guilt.
- Stop being a spectator. Don't stand on the outside watching what's going on (with your partner). Become *involved* in what's happening. Lose yourself in the emotion, fun and passion of the moment.
- Replace the negative thought lurking at the back of your mind (you know, the one that goes something like, *my sexual needs aren't important*) with a positive one.

Here are some examples of positive thoughts. Try saying these out loud and see how you feel.

## positive thoughts
### about my sexual needs

- I have a right to express my sexual needs.
- Being aroused and having orgasms is part of who I can be. It's important for me to be me during sex.
- My sexual needs are as important as the sexual needs of others.
- Focusing on my sexual needs is the way to being more aroused—it doesn't make me selfish.

If these are hard to say, try to figure out why. But keep saying the positive thoughts, anyway. It may simply be that talking like this feels odd because it's unfamiliar to you.

---

Well, you have to admit, these thoughts aren't the kind of thing you hear every day.

---

You're right, and more's the pity. If they were I probably wouldn't need to write this book. Anyway, just because you don't see them plastered all over billboards doesn't mean they shouldn't be! Now, there's a good idea . . . mmm.

However, repeating these thoughts over and over in your head will probably have the same effect. They'll become easier to hear and to accept.

The next step is to begin the Couple Change Program. Make sure you remember these positive thoughts. Say them before you start the program to put you in the right frame of mind. If necessary, repeat them to yourself *during* the program exercises.

ℚ

NOW, SOME OF you will try too hard to please a partner because of a fear that you aren't good enough as a lover and partner.

You probably worry about being judged by your partner and take this worry into your sexual activities. This, dear reader, will most definitely be a turn-off. Having an orgasm may be fine on your own or with someone you don't feel is important. It may be near impossible with a special partner who means a lot to you.

---

That I know only too well. But I can't help comparing myself with his ex-wife, who sounds so much more talented than I am. What do I do about that?

---

Let's take it bit by bit. Firstly, you need to decide if your fear of being judged is real or not. Perhaps your partner criticizes you a lot, in and out of bed. Naturally, you'll start comparing yourself with others (his ex-wife?), become tense, and wait for the next criticism. The last thing you'll be able to do is to lose yourself in the passion and emotions. You'll be a spectator, alert for any attack that may come your way. What you have is a relationship problem, not a sexual problem. I suggest you turn to chapter 11 (Making Relationship Changes) for further help in this area.

Perhaps your partner's criticism is about the way you express yourself sexually. He or she may have some particular sexual need that you don't feel comfortable with. Or it may be that he or she has asked you to become more sexually adventurous, more talkative about your problems, more affectionate, more sexually active, and so on—and has become frustrated at the lack of change. This frustration can easily lead to criticism if the two of you aren't able to talk through the differences between you.

This also suggests some difficulties in your relationship, so chapter 11 may be helpful for you, too.

What if there's no real reason for your fear of being judged by your partner? Perhaps your partner is loving and supportive, but you feel insecure and worry that he or she won't like you. This suggests that you have low self-esteem or negative feelings about yourself. You probably don't like yourself very much and so can't believe that your partner really wants to be with you.

If this fits you and you see the need to change the way you feel about yourself, I suggest you see a psychologist or do a course on improving self-esteem.

When you feel more positive and can truly believe the following phrase,

**I am a likable person,**

. . . move on to the Couple Change Program.

# 10

# doing it differently
## changing sexual practices

I T'S AMAZING HOW simple changes in the way we act sexually can help us to reach orgasm more easily. Don't be fooled, though. Our bodies may take a little while to adapt to new styles of doing things, no matter how simple they appear to be.

## lacking enough information about sexual arousal

IF YOU DON'T understand how your body becomes highly aroused, there's a good chance you'll experience orgasm difficulties. Information about arousal can come from reading books and other material, feedback from lovers, sex education classes, trying different approaches during masturbation or sex with a partner, and so on. Getting good information, however, is not easy.

Think back to the things you were taught at home or at school. You probably learned something about menstruation and pregnancy (and, then again, many women don't even receive this education). But what information were you given about orgasms? Or about getting aroused? Or about NOT getting aroused? At a guess, I'd say very little.

———————

Are you kidding? Even our sex education teacher avoided talking about the pleasure side of sexuality.

———————

Unfortunately, this is very common. There seems to be a problem in admitting that sex can be enjoyable, and that arousal and orgasms are part of this. Perhaps some educators assume that getting turned on is a "natural" reaction, so no one has to learn how to do it. Even many of the existing books on sexuality don't cover the topic of arousal and orgasm adequately. Given the lack of information on this topic, it's surprising that *every* woman doesn't have an orgasm problem.

Hopefully, this book has filled any gaps in your understanding of sexual arousal. But don't be afraid to read other books on sexuality. Learn as much as you can. Open your mind to ideas, even if you don't agree with them. After all, you always have the choice about which information to accept or reject.

Do you feel nervous about going into a bookstore and buying a book or magazine on sexuality? Many women do. If this is a problem, you can always place an order over the phone. The bookstore will then send it to you by mail. Many bookstores are also available on the Internet. By going to their Web sites, you can check out the books available and then order the ones that appeal to you.

Of course, actually going into a bookstore and browsing through the different books can be fun, so you might want to take a deep breath and go into the shop, *anyway*. Don't forget to tell yourself there's absolutely *nothing* to be ashamed or embarrassed about. Give yourself a pat on the back for having the courage to enter the door.

So much for the book learning. What about the real-life-experience learning? You can't beat this if you need to find out what kind of touch or situation lets you become highly aroused. If you've never learned about your own arousal, the hands-on approach is important.

It's also necessary if your arousal pattern has changed (e.g., from menopause, a spinal injury, or medical problems), and you need to find new ways of getting turned on. Women who feel ready to become less inhibited sexually will also find real-life-experience learning helpful in teaching them new ways of getting aroused.

The Personal Change Program will give you real-life-experience learning. It will teach you which kinds of touch and conditions can lead you to high levels of arousal. If you have a partner who wants to learn how to do this too, the Couple Change Program should be just what you need.

You should also take some time to reread the section in chapter 6 on *turn-on, turn-off patterns*. If you didn't complete the exercise, Identifying Your Turn-On and Turn-Off Patterns (page 111), do it now.

Like everyone else, you have a particular set of sexual triggers that can turn your sexual feelings on or off. It's important that you know what these triggers are. For example, you may need low lighting and a romantic atmosphere to get into a sexual mood. Or, your sexual feelings may completely disappear if you're not warm enough (or cool enough, if you're a woman having hot flashes/flushes).

You also need to know which kinds of touch and conditions help you to become highly aroused. For example, having your partner talk about sexual fantasies may begin to get you sexually excited, but you may need a quiet setting to become *highly* aroused.

Have you been trying to get aroused in a situation that doesn't include your sexual triggers? Check it out. Go back over your Turn-On/Turn-Off lists and put a cross X next to any Turn-Ons that are missing when you're trying to get highly aroused and to orgasm.

Ask yourself why they're missing. Do they have to be missing? Can the situation be changed so that your needs *are* met? Do you have the confidence or knowhow to make this happen?

Make a note in the box below (or in your notebook) of what you can change.

## the changes I *can* make

(so that the sexual situation includes my sexual triggers for high arousal)

1. _____

2. _____

3. _____

4. _____

Now make a list of what you *can't* change.

## the changes I *can't* make
to the sexual situation

1. _____

2. _____

3. _____

4. _____

Compare the two boxes. Will the changes that are *possible* for you to make be enough to help you become highly aroused? If yes, then make these changes as soon as possible. If they involve your partner, make sure you talk with him or her about this. If not, you may find it useful to talk over your situation with a psychologist or sexual therapist.

# fantasies that affect arousal |

DID YOU IDENTIFY a fantasy (or fantasies) that may be affecting your sexual arousal? Good for you! This isn't always easy to do (or admit to).

As you'll have learned earlier in this book, a fantasy that affects your arousal is likely to have two main characteristics. Firstly, it's a favorite one that you use most of the time. And, secondly, it involves people or activities that are quite different from your partner (or partners), or from what you usually do in a sexual situation.

By using a fantasy continuously, you'll condition your body to get turned on *only* to the kinds of people or activities in the fantasy. And if those people or activities are quite different from your own sexual situation, eventually it'll become hard to get highly aroused without using the favorite fantasy to boost your feelings of sexual pleasure. This, in turn, makes the fantasy even more important. And so, the whole problem keeps on going.

Fortunately, there are some steps you can take to change this situation.

## STEP 1

You must first decide whether you *want* to change your style of fantasizing. Although this may sound odd, the fact is that some women don't want to give up their fantasies. The reason is quite simple:

**a.** fantasies lead to feelings of sexual pleasure;

**b.** sexual pleasure can be rather addictive; in other words, we enjoy it and want it to continue;

**c.** since favorite fantasies tend to give us stronger feelings of sexual pleasure, it's hard to think about giving up or changing these fantasies.

If this fits you, yet you want to stop your fantasy from affecting your arousal, try focusing on the negative, *not* the positive, aspects of the fantasy. Your thinking should go something like this:

**a.** my fantasy seems to interfere with my getting highly aroused with my partner/any partner;

**b.** this is very frustrating for me and I want to be able to orgasm with my partner;

**c.** nothing will change unless I alter the way I fantasize.

---

But, last year I tried to cut out my fantasy. . . . I could
see the effect it was having. But then I lost ALL
sexual feelings. It wasn't much fun, I can tell you!

---

Yes, I can see how you wouldn't be keen to have another go at changing your fantasy. However, you may have tried the "cold-turkey" method (suddenly stopping), and this didn't work for you. I'll suggest another way in a moment.

But, first, it's important to realize that, for a few weeks, while you make changes to your fantasy, there *will* be a drop in your arousal level. After all, your body's been quite conditioned to one way of getting turned on. It can't make an overnight switch.

**So *be patient* and allow yourself enough time. Your body has to learn a different way of becoming aroused.**

It's hard for me to say how long this will take, because every woman is different. If you follow the exercises I'm about to describe, you should allow *at least* six weeks for change to occur (but, remember, it could take longer).

If you feel quite reluctant to give up your old fantasy, think about why this might be so. Perhaps the fantasy is telling you what you *really* want to be doing sexually, and your present sex life simply doesn't measure up. For example, you may be attracted to women and fantasize about them, but have a male partner, to whom you're less attracted (and with whom you're less likely to feel highly aroused).

If you want to stay with your fantasy, you have a choice. You can stay in your current situation and accept that the orgasm difficulties you have will continue. Or you can change your situation (your partner, what you do, how you do it) to look more like your fantasy.

## STEP 2

If you *do* want to change the fantasy, read on.

Take some time to think about what you could use in place of your troublesome fantasy. *Plan alternative fantasies* (remembering that at this point they won't seem as exciting as the old one). Aim to use more than one new fantasy (this is *very* important). Include a mixture of stories, people, and sexual activities. And *avoid* elements of the old fantasy (definitely!).

If you're having difficulty with this step, think about movies you've seen or books you've read. Take whatever time you need to develop interesting replacement fantasies. There's no point rushing to the next step with a new half-baked fantasy.

Once you've done this, find two positive statements to make about the new fantasies. Write these below or in your notebook, so that you won't forget them.

## positive statements
### about my new fantasies

1. _____

2. _____

3. _____

4. _____

If the thought of changing the old fantasy makes you feel anxious, I suggest you see a psychologist, who can help you to understand which element of the old fantasy seems to be affecting you this way.

## STEP 3

There are two ways of changing fantasies: **"cold turkey"** and **"fantasy swapping."** Both methods are equally effective, but some women find one method easier than the other. Keep an open mind, and start by choosing the one that appeals to you most. If this doesn't suit you, then try the other.

Both methods are best done while masturbating. This allows you to concentrate, without interruption, on the changes you're trying to make.

If you can't handle the idea of masturbation (but read chapter 13 before you finish with this subject), then include the exercises described below during sexual activity with your partner. It would help to warn your partner of the temporary drop in your arousal levels (but if he or she doesn't know about the "problem fantasy," you'll have to figure out how to get around that one).

Let me now show you how to do each method during masturbation. These exercises can be combined with the Personal Change Program.

### Cold-turkey method

1. With this strategy, you immediately stop using the old fantasy. The new replacement fantasies should be used, keeping in mind that your body will need time to adjust to the change.
2. If possible, you should masturbate two or three times a week for at least six weeks (but take as long as you need), using the new fantasies. If you can't do the exercise this often, be prepared for a longer adjustment time.
3. Remember to stay positive about the new fantasies. If you find yourself thinking negatively during the exercise, *immediately* switch your thinking to the positive statements you identified earlier in this section (*Positive statements about my new fantasies*). Remind yourself why you're making these changes.

### Fantasy-swapping method

1. Begin masturbating with the old fantasy for about one minute. Then switch to the new fantasy for at least three minutes. The longer you can go with the new fantasy, the better.
2. If you feel your arousal die away, return to the old fantasy for another minute. Then, once again, switch to the new one. Stay with this for another three minutes. Keep this pattern going until you wish to finish.
3. *Always, always* end your masturbation session with the *new* fantasy.

**4.** Do this two or three times a week for at least eight weeks (but take as long as you need). As in the "cold-turkey" method, keep your thoughts positive.

Regardless of the method you use, don't even think about orgasms at this point. It will be a while before you can reach high enough levels of arousal for this to happen. Keep in mind that changing your fantasies is a step towards overcoming your orgasm difficulties.

If you're finding the exercise difficult, see a sexual therapist, who can help to identify what the problem is.

# habits that affect arousal |

SOME SEXUAL HABITS can make it difficult for us to reach high levels of sexual arousal. For example, if you orgasm during masturbation with one kind of touch (perhaps using a vibrator or pressing against a hard bench), it may be extremely difficult to have an orgasm with your partner if he or she can't copy this kind of contact.

We can easily develop sexual habits by doing the same sexual activity over and over again. This can condition you to get aroused only when you do that activity. Other types of lovemaking will then leave you cold (or at least lukewarm).

It's easy to understand how this happens. The pleasure of orgasm acts as a very powerful "reward." It encourages us to continue doing whatever it is that will lead to this feeling of pleasure. If we regularly do the same thing to reach orgasm, our body learns to prefer this method. Sexual habits are often developed during masturbation, but can also be formed during sex with a partner.

If you believe you may have sexual habits that stop you from having an orgasm, look at the questions I ask in the *Sexual Habits* quizzes on the next two pages.

# my sexual habits
(when on my own)

1. Do you use exactly the same sexual activity, position, or touch each time?

              Yes ☐    No ☐

   When did you start doing this? _____

2. What happens to your level of arousal if you try another kind of activity, position, or touch?

   _____

   _____

3. Does the activity, position, or touch you prefer during masturbation get used during sex with a partner?
   If not, why?

              Yes ☐    No ☐

   Is it too difficult to copy?

              Yes ☐    No ☐

4. If you try new ways of being sexual, do you find it difficult to get aroused, even though you're keen to experiment?

              Yes ☐    No ☐

If you don't masturbate, you can still condition your arousal patterns by doing the same thing each time you have sexual activity with a partner.

Answer the questions that follow:

## my sexual habits
(with a partner)

**1.** Do you use exactly the same sexual activity,     Yes     No
position or touch each time?                      ❐     ❐

When did you start doing this? _____

**2.** What happens to your level of arousal if you try another
kind of activity, position, or touch when you're with a partner?

_____

_____

**3.** Do you get angry if your partner wants     Yes     No
you to try to get aroused in a different way?    ❐     ❐

Take some time to think over these questions. Be honest with
yourself. From your answers see if you can identify:

- whether the range of sexual activities, positions and touch
  that arouse you is narrow or wide
- whether there is a difference between what you need to get
  highly aroused and what happens between you and your
  partner. In other words, is there a gap between what actually occurs sexually (the reality) and what you've conditioned yourself to be aroused to (the habit)?

Did you decide that the range of activities that turn you on is narrow? And that it's hard for a partner to copy what you need to get
highly aroused?

If so, you may want to expand your range to make it easier to
orgasm. The best way to do this is to begin with developing your
masturbation style (see the program on the next page). Later you
can take the changes into your sexual activities with a partner. You

may find it helpful to combine the exercises I've given below with the Personal Change Program and, later, the Couple Change Program.

If you're unhappy with masturbating, you could attempt to make the changes during sexual activity with your partner. However, some sexual habits can be difficult to shift in this way, and you may have to spend more time doing the exercise before getting the results you want.

## STEP 1

As in the previous section, it's important to make sure you really want to change your sexual habits. There's no point starting with a half-hearted approach. We both know that won't work. If you aren't interested in changing, be honest with yourself as to why this is so. Perhaps you're not prepared to give up the old ways. Perhaps this isn't a good time to be making changes. If you're lacking in enthusiasm, this is probably a sign that you're not ready for change.

## STEP 2

Decide how you would like to change the way you masturbate. Read books, ask friends, or simply use your imagination. Think of several different kinds of sexual activity, touch, and positions to use. Make sure you choose ways of arousing yourself that can be easily copied by a partner.

For example, if your habit has been to squeeze your legs together to get aroused, you may be aware of how hard this is to copy when with a partner. You'll need to choose a new masturbation style that allows you to get turned on with your legs apart.

Another example: if you've always used a vibrator and now want to learn to be aroused by fingers or a softer, less-regular touch, you'll need to choose ways of touching that are more gentle and varied.

At this point, find a couple of positive statements to make about the new styles you've chosen. This is important. There's no use try-ing something new if all the time you're hating what you're doing. Write your positive statements on the next page.

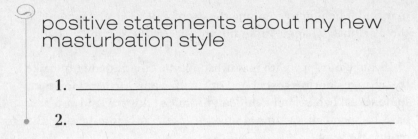

## positive statements about my new masturbation style

1. _____

2. _____

### STEP 3

You can choose between the **"cold-turkey"** or **"style-swapping"** methods to help you make the change.

#### Cold-turkey method

1. First, *ban* yourself from using the old masturbation style. Practice with the new methods two to three times a week, for at least six weeks.
2. Resist going back to your old style; it may be hard to get aroused for several weeks (maybe even months), but be patient. Eventually, your body will begin to adapt to the new methods.
3. Make sure your thoughts about the new method stay positive. Use the positive statements written in the previous box to help you do this. There's no point wishing you were using your old style. Remember to breathe nice and easily. You want to stay relaxed.

#### Style-swapping method

1. Begin masturbation with the old style for one minute, then switch to the new one for at least three minutes (but go for as long as you wish). If your arousal starts to die away, return to the old style for one minute, before switching again to the new method.
2. Continue this pattern until you decide to finish. But, *always, always* finish with the new style.
3. Do this two to three times a week, for at least eight weeks (but you may need longer). Stay focused on the positive aspects of the new method. Say your positive statements to help you do this. Stay relaxed.

Whichever method you use, don't worry about orgasms. Just concentrate on making the switch to a new way of being aroused. Later, your arousal level will get stronger as your body adapts to the change.

Remember, the old way blocked your arousal from building to orgasm levels. Remind yourself that it takes time to make changes. You've been practicing the old way for _____ years (you can fill in the length of time), so don't expect instant miracles.

If you're having problems, head off to a sexual therapist, who can help you work through the program I've just outlined.

## orgasm during vaginal intercourse |

THERE'S A BIG difference between *wanting* to enjoy orgasm during vaginal intercourse and feeling you *should* have an orgasm during intercourse. Unfortunately, it's the last of these that affect many women. They:

- feel pressured to have an orgasm during intercourse
- feel a failure if they don't orgasm during intercourse
- assume that orgasm should happen during intercourse
- believe that orgasms felt during non-intercourse activities (e.g., oral sex, using hands, rubbing bodies) aren't as acceptable as orgasms during intercourse
- believe that during intercourse both people should orgasm together

Each of these regrettable ideas puts pressure on women to have an orgasm. And, as you know, dear reader, *that* is the last thing you need if you want to reach high arousal levels.

So, take a moment to check whether your desire to have an orgasm during vaginal intercourse comes from the thought that you

SHOULD ...
MUST ...
HAVE TO ...

If any of these words fit you, then stop and ask yourself, *Why do I think this way? Is there a real pressure on me to orgasm during intercourse or is it imagined?*

If it's a real pressure coming from your partner, see if you can find out why he's doing this. Does he think this is the "right" way for women to orgasm? Or, is it something else?

---

> The problem is, he thinks he's failed as a lover if I don't orgasm. Sometimes I fake it just to make him feel better.

---

Many men seem to think this way. Remember, their sex education is no better at tackling the topic of women's orgasms than our own. This means *you* have to teach him. Perhaps getting him to read this book would be a good place to start. Don't forget, though, to talk to him about the ways in which you prefer to have an orgasm.

If the belief that you should have an orgasm during intercourse is coming from you, rather than others, then you're putting the pressure on yourself. Think about why you do this. Check whether you're prepared to change the way you think. Remind yourself that many, many women do *not* have an orgasm during intercourse.

In fact, having an orgasm *before* or *after* intercourse is preferred by many women. Why? Because they can then focus on their own sexual pleasure without worrying about their partner's needs. They can also choose to have an orgasm in the way they enjoy most.

So, stop worrying about trying to have an orgasm during intercourse. Enjoy the ways you *do* orgasm.

However, if you'd like to orgasm during intercourse simply because this will give you pleasure, then read on. Otherwise, skip the next section *without* guilt. You don't have an orgasm difficulty just because you prefer to orgasm during sexual activity that isn't vaginal intercourse.

☙

MANY WOMEN FIND they can't orgasm during intercourse because their arousal levels stay too low (or drop too low). This situation usually occurs when the glans, hood, and shaft of their clitoris are not being touched by their partner's body in the way that builds their arousal. In some intercourse positions, these areas may not be touched at all.

Some inner areas of the clitoris (the legs, the bulbs, the urethral sponge, and perineal sponge) are probably stimulated by intercourse, but, for many women, this won't be enough to make the entire clitoris fully erect. It seems that the glans and shaft need to be touched for full swelling to occur. When the erectile tissue of the clitoris is fully erect, an orgasm is more likely to be triggered.

Once you understand what's happening, it can be relatively easy to make changes so that orgasm can occur. I have some simple suggestions you may want to try.

Firstly, engage in sex in other ways that you like until you're *quite* sexually aroused. Then begin having intercourse. With your arousal already high, it should be easier to reach the levels needed to orgasm.

Secondly, create and keep high levels of sexual arousal by touching the glans and shaft of your clitoris (through the hood) during intercourse with your fingers. You can also have your partner do this. Of course, you'll need to tell him when you want to be touched. Don't expect him to be a mind reader—especially in the middle of his own sexual pleasure.

Another way to keep your arousal high is to use intercourse positions that allow you to press the glans and shaft of your clitoris against your partner's body in a way that is stimulating.

Try different intercourse positions, and discover which ones allow you to follow these suggestions. The most likely positions are those where the woman is on top (sitting or lying) and the scissor position, where the man is lying to the side with his legs between the woman's. Don't put too much attention on *thinking* about what you're doing; otherwise, you may lose your arousal altogether. Just relax and enjoy yourself. It may take a while to learn these skills, but what's the rush? If you continue to have difficulty, see a sexual therapist.

I should also mention that physical conditions such as weak pelvic muscles can sometimes play a part in making it difficult for a woman to orgasm during intercourse. If you have any doubts, see a doctor with experience in the sexual area.

◡

BEFORE I FINISH, let me say something about simultaneous orgasms. Some women try to have orgasms at the same time as their partner. They think this is the best way to have intercourse. The fact is, it's very difficult climbing up the arousal hill at exactly the same speed as your partner. Trying to do this can be distracting and result in your being turned *off*, not on. The truth is that many couples don't climax together without a great deal of experience. Take care that you don't add *this* pressure to any others you feel. Otherwise, you may end up with no orgasm at all.

## undoing the effects of sexual abuse |

WOMEN WHO HAVE been sexually attacked or abused often find it difficult to build arousal. Their own arousal can remind them of the sexual arousal of their attacker/abuser. Sometimes it's the sexual arousal of a partner that triggers these memories.

> That seems to fit me. I really trust my partner but,
> during sex, before I can stop myself, I'm thinking
> back to those horrible memories of being forced into
> doing sexual things when I was thirteen. You can
> imagine what that does to my sexual feelings. . . .

Yes, you wouldn't stay aroused for very long. As soon as those memories come to mind, you'll probably have negative thoughts and then feel upsetting emotions to match. Before you realize what's happening, your feelings of sexual pleasure will be replaced by negativity. Instead of climbing the arousal hill, you'll be sliding back down to the bottom at a very fast pace.

To stop this happening, you'll need to break the connection between the memory of the sexual abuse or attack and the sexual pleasure you or your partner feel. Fortunately, there are ways of doing this. Let me show you how.

## STEP 1

First of all, check how motivated you are to think about your past abuse. If you've previously discussed what happened with a therapist or friend, you may feel ready to focus on the effects it's had on your sexual feelings.

On the other hand, thinking about these past experiences may still make you very upset. If this situation fits you, it may not be the time to work on your orgasm difficulties. Before beginning my Programs, wait until you feel emotionally stronger or get professional help. Having said that, I should add that some women find the Programs actually help them to work through their feelings about the sexual abuse or attack.

Read through the steps I've outlined below and decide for yourself if you're ready to move on.

## STEP 2

Many sexually abused women find they become tense when they first begin to get turned on. Others don't react this way until their feelings begin to build towards orgasm.

This tension is often a sign of anxiety or fear. Many women feel themselves stiffen in readiness for an imagined attack. Because of the past abuse or attack experiences, they link sexual arousal with the need to protect themselves. The tension they experience can happen quickly and without their having time to consciously think about past events.

**If your body is tense and you're filled with fear or anxiety, it's going to be very difficult to stay sexually aroused.**

That being the case, let's talk about what you can do to stop that tension.

First, let's try to identify the different parts of your reaction. Remember, there's a link between thoughts and emotions.

1. Your reaction probably starts with negative thoughts (about being unsafe).
2. These thoughts will lead to your feeling negative emotions (fear, anxiety, discomfort, and so on).

**3.** Your muscles then tighten as you imagine being attacked or abused again.

**4.** You become swamped by this negativity and switch off from sexual pleasure. The result is **orgasmic meltdown!**

---

Well, I'm not aware of any negative thoughts. My whole body just seems to react.

---

Many women feel exactly the same way. Sometimes, the reactions happen so quickly that it appears as if no thoughts have occurred.

However, trying to identify the negative thoughts that stop your sexual arousal from building more strongly is an important first step to change. With a little concentration and time, it's often possible to do it.

I want you to take some time *now* to try to identify the negative thoughts that come into your mind during sex. Find somewhere private and quiet where you won't be interrupted for five minutes. Shut your eyes and picture the times when your sexual arousal has shut down. It's easier to do this if it's happened recently. Try to remember the emotions you felt as this happened. See if you can identify any thoughts that may have popped into your mind just before these emotions came to the surface.

If this isn't possible, don't worry. Wait until you're involved in some *actual* sexual activity and can notice what's happening. As soon as you feel yourself switch off, STOP what you're doing and ask yourself,

**What was I thinking about a moment ago?**

Sometimes it's easier to catch the thought when it happens rather than later when you're not feeling aroused. If you're with a partner, don't forget to tell him or her what you're doing. Say you need to lie quietly for a moment while you concentrate on what just happened.

If you identify the negative thoughts, write them in the box below.

## negative thoughts
that pop into my head when I'm turned on

_____

_____

_____

_____

Once you've identified the negative thoughts that seem to make
you switch off, go to Step 3.

What if you can't pick up any thoughts? There may be a good reason for this. You may have learned to make your mind go blank during the experience of sexual abuse or attack. It would have been a
smart way of blocking out the horror of what was happening. This
strategy of shutting out all thoughts and feelings may have carried
over into sexual situations that _aren't_ abusive. You may find yourself
blanking out during sex (either on your own or with a partner).
When this happens, it will be difficult to "hear" the thoughts that
make you switch off.

Let me see if I can help you to stop this blocking of your
thoughts. But, first let me say: you must be patient with yourself.
These changes can take a little time. Try the suggestions I give you,
but don't pressure yourself. You need to feel ready to hear what your
mind has to "say."

Begin by asking yourself the following question (both during sex
and at other times):

**Question:**
_If I weren't blanking out my mind right now, what might I be thinking
about my sexual feelings?_

Try to imagine what your mind might be thinking about. Don't worry if the thoughts you get don't seem logical. They don't have to be. You may find the words that come into your mind are those of a frightened child, rather than an adult. Avoid judging yourself for being like this. It's a natural reaction in this situation.

Some examples of thoughts that might be lurking in your mind during sex are:

- *Why doesn't he leave me alone?*
- *I'd better be careful.*
- *If I lie still, it'll soon be over.*
- *It's wrong to like my sexy feelings.*
- *I can't do anything, I have to suffer it.*
- *I'm scared I'll get hurt.*
- *This feels like when I was abused.*
- *I shouldn't be enjoying myself like this.*

Once you've identified your negative thoughts, move on to Step 3. Don't worry if you're having trouble doing Step 2. Keep trying, and remember what I said: be patient. See a therapist if you'd like further help.

## STEP 3

Now, let's consider the negative thoughts that came up during sex. Not very encouraging, are they? Can you see how they would lead to negative emotions? And to your body tightening up?

You're caught in a vicious circle. Your negative reactions reinforce the idea that sex isn't any fun. And if it isn't fun, you won't want to continue feeling sexual pleasure. You *definitely* won't be interested in getting aroused enough to orgasm.

To break this vicious circle, you'll need to begin with the thoughts. Negative thoughts need to be changed into positive ones.

---

I don't understand. Nothing I think or do is going to change what happened to me in the past, is it?

---

You're absolutely right!

**You can't change what happened in the past—but you CAN change the way you react right now.**

Although changing over to positive thoughts about your present life may seem difficult, it can make a difference. Let me give you some examples of positive thoughts that can be said in place of negative ones:

## swapping negative thoughts for positive ones

- I'm now safe; my partner is loving and trustworthy.
- I can relax and enjoy myself sexually; this has nothing to do with the past.
- It's okay for me to let myself get aroused; this is a safe situation, and I can take control if I need to.

Take some time *right now* to think about which positive thoughts will suit you. You don't have to use the examples I've given. However, just make sure the positive thoughts you use include the following messages:

- **message 1:** The past and the present are not the same.
- **message 2:** The present can be safe and enjoyable.
- **message 3:** You can take control of the present if you need.

If you've decided on some positive thoughts of your own, write them in the box below.

## my positive thoughts

1. _____

2. _____

3. _____

4. _____

If you need help with this, see an experienced therapist before moving on to the next stage.

## STEP 4

Now that you've identified some positive thoughts, the next step is to apply them when you most need them—during sex.

First, say them at times when you're *not* having sex. Say them at least three times a day for a week. Listen carefully to what you're saying. The more you say them in this way, the more you'll begin to believe them. Don't just rattle the words off, parrot fashion. This won't change anything. Continue saying your positive statements until they become part of your thinking.

Now, let's take them into the sexual situation. Before you begin sexual activity, repeat your positive statements a couple of times to yourself. As you become aroused, be ready to use them *any time you find yourself switching off.* Don't focus too much on the negative thoughts. Just notice when they pop into your head, then immediately switch to your positive thoughts.

Add: *Relax, everything's fine* at the end of each positive thought. Take some deep breaths to help you along.

Keep doing this and, gradually, you'll feel your body reacting differently. Don't worry if this takes some weeks. Remember, you're retraining your mind, emotions, and body. These things can't be changed in a day, no matter how much you'd like them to be!

If you're doing this while having sex with your partner, try telling him or her what's happening. You need to get support for the changes you're attempting. This is more likely to happen if you share your experiences at the time, rather than clamming up.

There are two ways in which you can use the Change Program I've just outlined. Firstly, you can try the four steps as I've described them here. Or, you could do Steps 1 to 3 now and then make Step 4 part of the Personal Change Program and Couple Change Program. Simply, follow each of these Programs as I outline them in chapters 13 and 14 and, if you find yourself reacting or thinking negatively, follow the suggestions I've just outlined in Step 4.

# 11

# making relationship changes

WE WOMEN ARE a sensitive lot. Our desire for sex and romance can be so easily dampened if relationships aren't going well. So, too, can feelings of sexual pleasure, which may disappear in seconds if we sense there's a problem with our partner.

For many women, this loss of arousal is temporary, and sexual feelings return when the relationship seems to be working smoothly again.

However, some relationship problems are not so easily overcome. In earlier chapters, I discussed four problems that interfere with women getting aroused enough to orgasm: resentment towards a partner, boredom with a partner, loss of physical attraction to a partner and difficulties in communicating sexual needs to a partner.

Some women may not even try to have sex when any of these situations exists. Others will begin sex, but soon find there's not enough sexual passion to carry them to orgasm.

Let me now talk about each of these issues and what you might be able to do to build your sexual arousal so that orgasm is possible.

## resentment towards a partner |

RESENTMENT TOWARDS YOUR partner is a passion killer, no doubt about that. Picture the scene. There you are, in the middle of lovemaking, and you start thinking about something your partner said or did that annoyed you. From that moment, the more he or she touches you, the more irritated you get.

What chance do you have of really enjoying your sexual pleasure in this situation? You guessed it—absolutely none! How can you? You've switched off. You're *thinking*, and *thinking negatively*. As a result, any sexual arousal you felt at the beginning will soon fade to nothing.

I don't have to tell you this. You KNOW exactly what's happening! The question is, what do you do about it?

Well, finding a way to feel happier with your partner is one obvious solution to your sexual difficulties.

---

Obvious, yes, but not always easy to do. How do I get rid of three years worth of resentment? There's no magic wand to make everything wonderful again.

---

No, there isn't. But, resentment may take less time to get rid of than it took to build up. Let's look at what your resentment is likely to be made up of:

- blaming your partner for what you see as some past wrongdoing (which may still be occurring)
- feeling upset at how this wrongdoing has affected you
- feeling you have no control over the situation
- thinking daily about your partner's past wrongdoing, which leaves you feeling constantly annoyed
- avoiding expressing the anger directly (perhaps you tried in the past without much luck)

That's a lot of negative thought and emotion that you feel *in the present* about *the past*. The problem is, while you're busy feeling so negative about the past, you may be missing some positive things that are happening in your life now.

Take a few moments right now to check out whether there's a nice side to your relationship. Do you have enough positive feelings towards your partner to want to give up your resentment? That's a tough question, isn't it? When you're so resentful, it can be hard to see the wood for the trees. If you've been looking at the negatives for a long time, the good parts of your relationship don't stand out too easily, do they?

Stop and think about what it would be like if you were no longer resentful. Would you still want to be with your partner? Do you still care for him or her, somewhere deep down inside? Is there still enough feeling to go on with the relationship?

I'm often amazed at how feelings of love and caring return when the resentment is removed. Women who were ready to move out find they can once again enjoy their partner's company.

Of course, this doesn't happen to everyone. Sometimes the resentment has been around for so long that it's destroyed any love that used to exist. What's left is the sense of caring that comes from having spent many years with a partner. But it's a "companionship" type of caring, not the feeling of being "lovers." And recognizing this shift from lover to companion can create further resentment . . . and so it goes.

If you feel no motivation to improve the relationship, the suggestions I am about to make won't interest you. You may want to think seriously, instead, about separating from your partner, or at least talk to a psychologist or relationship therapist about your feelings.

If you're keen to see the relationship improve, you may still want to head off to a therapist. It's often easier to have a trained professional help you through the issues.

In the meantime, let me make some suggestions that may help in shifting your resentment.

## SUGGESTION #1

Let the past be in the past. If there's something happening in your relationship *now* that you're angry about, deal with that. Stick to whatever it is that's annoying you *right now*. Don't drag up the past, even if the issue you're annoyed with at the moment has occurred before. Be clear about what is making you annoyed and what changes you want. Keep your comments short and simple. Don't go on and on. Otherwise, the point you're making will only get lost in all those words.

## SUGGESTION #2

Make a list of what you need *right now* to be happier/happy in your relationship. Get your partner to make a similar list. Make sure the lists are quite specific. Don't make general statements such as, *I need more love, I want you to be more responsible.* What does that mean? Your partner may interpret these words differently from you, and then there'll be *more* resentment. Be specific. Be clear. For example, *I would like you to give me a hug each morning before you go to work, or I would like you to organize some of our social outings.* These statements say clearly what it is you want.

The next step is to discuss each item on the lists to see if each of you is prepared to meet the other's requests. With a therapist, if possible, work through these lists (taking one from your list, then one from your partner's list . . . until you finish). A trained professional can often prevent you from getting stuck in the same old arguments.

If you want to try this without any help, stick closely to Suggestion #1. Don't make demands or get into blaming the other. Yes, I know this is easier said than done, but simply try to say what you need to be happy. Then ask your partner if he or she is able to oblige. If you're both prepared to try to meet the other's needs, there's a good chance your relationship will improve.

## SUGGESTION #3

If you do have sex with your partner, recognize that thinking negatively about him or her during sex will turn you off. If negative thoughts pop into your head, immediately switch to positive ones. Remember what it is you like about your partner and your relationship. And don't forget to focus on the positive aspects of the sexual situation you're in. Relax and enjoy your sexual arousal.

By the way, try to remember that your resentment is stopping *you* from enjoying sex and having an orgasm. Seems a shame, doesn't it?

You may find it helpful to carry out the first two suggestions before trying the third.

SUGGESTION #4

When you feel *less* resentful towards your partner, you may consider doing the Couple Change Program. This can help to bring you closer. It's also a good way to begin having sex again, if you're feeling distant from your partner and don't know how to get the closeness back into your relationship.

# boredom with a partner |

LET'S TAKE A few moments to try to understand your boredom a little better. Be as honest as you can with the following quiz. There's no point trying to fool yourself.

## boredom with a partner quiz

1. How long have you felt bored with your partner?

   _____

   _____

2. Did something happen to make you feel this way?

   _____

   _____

3. Are you bored with your partner *as a person in general* or *as a sexual partner?*

   _____

   _____

4. If you're bored with your partner in general, what *qualities* about him or her bore you?

_____

_____

5. If you're bored with your partner sexually, what does he or she *do* that bores you?

_____

_____

6. What's missing that would make the relationship exciting?

_____

_____

Hopefully, these questions have helped you to pinpoint where your boredom is coming from. Now, try the next three questions:

## question 1:
### do you want to remain in the relationship? why?

_____

_____

For some women, admitting they're bored with their partner as a person or sexually can be enough to consider separating. They shudder at the thought of being with the same partner for the next ten years. Others are prepared to tolerate the situation, but have plenty of interesting friends and interests to make life attractive.

## question 2:
### have you thought of saying something? if not, why?

_____

_____

Many women haven't. Because they're afraid of hurting their partner, they keep the problem to themselves. If asked about their difficulties with orgasm, they mutter something about being tired and then change the subject.

> Yeah, I've done that. But he's really a nice guy. He tries hard and is a good father and husband.

And it's really important to remember all these positive qualities. Yet, unless you're prepared to let him know what _you_ need to be happier sexually (or generally), resentment will eventually build.

> Well, I suppose it has already. I get annoyed that he can't see how boring sex has become.

Perhaps he _has_—and is afraid to say anything to _you_. Perhaps you're both so scared of rocking the boat that nothing will ever change. This leads me to the last question you need to ask yourself.

## question 3:
### do you believe something could be changed?

_____

_____

Would your partner listen to why you're having trouble with sex-ual arousal? Can you be assertive enough to explain your feelings and say what would make sex more exciting for you?

You could begin by making a list of how you'd like sex to be different. Be honest and clear. Don't attack or blame.

Next, tell your partner that you have something you'd like to talk about. Make a time to meet when you're both free and when there'll be no interruptions. Don't wait until it's late at night and you're tired.

If your partner wants to know what it's about, simply say you aren't as happy with sex as you used to be and you'd like to have a chat about this. You might add that you'd be interested in whether your partner has similar feelings. (You could even ask your partner to make a list of how he or she would like sex to be different.)

Show your partner the list you made earlier. Say how hard it is to talk about this topic, and mention your fear of hurting him or her. Try to find out whether your partner feels the same. Now, make a joint list of what you'd both like *and would be happy to try*. There's no point including something that either of you would really dislike.

At this stage you don't have to feel entirely comfortable with each item on your joint list. New activities and new ways of doing things sometimes make us feel a bit awkward at first. In time, however, they can become enjoyable.

You may find the Couple Change Program helpful in overcom-ing your awkwardness. Follow the program as outlined in chapter 14 and, when you get to the last step, simply add anything else you'd like to try. By then you should be ready to experiment.

Remember, change isn't going to just happen (no magic wands, I'm afraid). And, with each passing month and year of boredom, your difficulties with orgasm are likely to get worse.

## loss of physical attraction |

REALIZING YOU'RE NO longer attracted to your partner may leave you with a sinking feeling. Many women start to think about separation and worry that they'll be unable to cope on their own. However, before you head down this track, take some time to identify exactly what's happened.

First, think about whether your partner has changed in appearance or not. Perhaps he or she has put on weight, or started to dress with less care than before. Maybe illness has left him or her looking thin and gray.

I know my partner's put on a lot of weight
since we met, but I feel pretty ashamed of myself
because I should feel attracted to her no matter
what she looks like.

Many women feel the same way, blaming themselves for what they judge to be shallowness. However, each of us has been conditioned to find a certain "look" attractive, and the truth is that it's hard to adjust to something different.

You may love your partner, but this doesn't keep you from being attracted to a different body shape, coloring or style of presentation.

What do you do, then, if your partner's appearance has changed? Well, first decide if the change is *permanent* or *temporary*. If it's a temporary situation, you may choose to wait out the change. You might tell your partner about why you're having orgasm difficulties. Often they've sensed the problem already and are relieved to talk openly about it.

If the change seems to be permanent, you need to think about the options available to you. Some women see a need to separate. Others take lovers from time to time. And some simply use fantasy to help them become aroused during sex with their partner.

If you need to talk through these different options with someone, a few sessions with an experienced therapist will probably be helpful. It can be a great relief to talk to someone who won't judge you.

❧

LET'S THINK ABOUT the other possibility: that your partner hasn't changed in appearance at all. What can this mean? Well, perhaps it's *you* who has changed.

Think about what turns you on. Has this changed since you first began expressing yourself sexually? Believe it or not, changes like this can happen. Perhaps the type of person, body, or presentation that was attractive to you when you were younger no longer turns you on. While this may be interesting (and even exciting), it can also be disturbing—especially if your partner fits the *old* turn-on image.

Once again, it's time to consider your options. You could go on as you are. You could finish the relationship. You could take a lover who is attractive to you. Or, you could use fantasy to help you become aroused with your present partner.

Another interesting option is to ask your partner to change his or her appearance, if possible, to match your attractions. Of course, this means you'll need to talk about the problem. This can be hard to do, but may help your partner to understand why you're unable to orgasm at the moment.

If you feel uncertain about what to do, make the time to speak to a therapist. Don't give up. The situation may not be as hopeless as you think.

## communicating sexual needs |

YOU MAY BE unable to orgasm easily simply because of a fear of saying what you need to build your arousal. This leads to a situation where your partner either gives up in frustration after some time of trying to turn you on, or pushes on regardless, valiantly trying to arouse you. If you're lucky, he or she will eventually figure it out.

---

Well, you can see that didn't happen.
Otherwise I wouldn't be reading this book for
some clues to my problem with orgasm!

---

True. But, reading this book suggests you're prepared to look at how *you* can do things differently. That's a better option than waiting for your partner to learn how to "read your mind."

With a little help, you could learn to speak up for yourself. Stop for a moment and think about why this is such a problem for you. Are you shy and find it difficult to voice your needs in any situation? Were you brought up to keep your views to yourself? Do you fear being rejected, criticized, laughed at? Are you worried you'll appear too eager? These are some of the reasons women avoid communicating their sexual needs.

The good news is that your difficulties with communicating are probably learned. With a little professional help, you should be able to *unlearn* them. It's worth talking to a psychologist or counselor about this. There are also many self-help books that teach women how to be more assertive.

Keep in mind that standing up for yourself also tells your partner that:

- your sexual needs are important
- your sexual needs are as important as theirs
- it's perfectly natural for you to focus on your sexual needs
- you don't expect your partner to be a mind reader about what turns you on

When you feel ready to talk to your partner, decide which would be the best way to do it. You might want to chat at a time when you're not having sex. On the other hand, it can be quite sexy telling your partner what you like while cuddled up in bed. You may even want to *show* your partner what you like.

This doesn't have to be too serious. Have fun with it. Have a few laughs. It won't be long before you feel comfortable talking about your sexual needs. In fact, it won't be long before you'll wonder what all the fuss was about.

# 12

# dealing with
## health factors

## pain during sex |

THERE ARE TWO kinds of pain that affect women's level of sexual arousal. The first is called *primary* pain: caused by an actual physical or medical condition that creates pain during sex (see Cause #16 for examples of this).

The second type of pain is known as *secondary* pain, and it occurs when the *fear* of pain during sex causes pain, rather than any medical or physical condition. How can this happen? It's quite simple. If you have a fear that sex will cause you pain, your body and mind quickly react. You'll become tense, tightening the muscles in your pelvis and genital area. This can make your skin quite sensitive to touch. You'll also become anxious and focus all your attention on the possibility of pain, rather than on sexual pleasure.

The result of all this is that you'll stop getting aroused. Rather than becoming wet and relaxed, you'll be tense, sensitive, and dry. Your focus will then turn to negative, rather than positive aspects of sex. Not surprisingly, all these reactions combine to make sexual contact uncomfortable and painful.

The fear of pain may come from:

- previous experiences when an actual physical or medical condition *did* cause pain during sex. Even when that condition no longer exists or gives you pain, it can be hard to break the habit of becoming tense and anxious when you have sexual contact.
- previous experiences that taught you sexual contact is likely to cause pain

---

> Hey, that fits me. My mother told me just before my
> wedding that it would hurt. I knew what she meant,
> all right. Well, then I was so nervous about feeling
> pain during intercourse that naturally it WAS
> painful—and has been ever since.

---

Not surprising, is it? Can you see the chain of events? Negative thinking (your mother's warning) led to you to feel anxious. This led to tightening of the muscles in your pelvis and around the entrance of your vagina. As you "waited" in fear for the pain, your lubrication or wetness stopped, leaving your genitals dry. In very little time, this led to real pain as your partner tried to enter your dry vagina.

I'm sure by now you probably tense up automatically when having intercourse (or maybe *any* kind of sex) and feel pain a lot of the time. You'll certainly have no interest in hanging around long enough to orgasm!

## DEALING WITH PAIN
### Primary pain

What can you do about the effects of pain on your sexual arousal? To begin with, let me talk about primary pain. The first step is to find out whether the cause of the pain can be removed or reduced. If you're not sure what the problem is, visit your doctor. If you don't feel comfortable talking to your regular doctor about your sexual arousal difficulties, go to someone else.

If the reason for the pain is identified and medication is available to treat and remove the condition, *do not have sex until you're healed.*

Do you see the reason for this? Pain during sex can quickly condition you to turn off your sexual arousal. So, the more you try sex that is painful, the more strongly you'll learn to switch *off* sexually. Obviously, you don't want to learn this lesson any more than you already have. So, stay clear of any sexual activity that creates pain until you're certain that the medical problem is gone. And don't forget to tell your partner what's going on.

When you no longer have the condition that caused the pain in the first place, then you will need to learn how to switch your feelings back on again. To learn how to orgasm once again on your own, use the Personal Change Program. It should help you to regain confidence in enjoying your sexual arousal without the expectation of pain. To regain your confidence with your partner, try the Couple Change Program.

What do you do if you can't get rid of the pain? There are several possibilities:

- Your doctor may be able to give you some pain-reducing medication to be used when you want to be sexual. Don't be embarrassed about asking for it. Remind yourself it's perfectly natural to want to enjoy sexual pleasure.
- You could experiment with what you do sexually, in order to find the activity or position that is *least* painful. As you become more aroused, stick with this activity or position. Changing to something that increases the pain will only make you anxious and increase your chance of feeling pain.
- If there's a particular time of the day when you're more likely to feel pain, avoid it. Plan sex around those times when you're experiencing the least amount of pain.
- Give yourself permission to stop sex when pain occurs and, if possible, start sex when the pain has gone. Don't push yourself beyond your limits. This will only set up negative feelings towards sex again.
- You could also try giving more attention to the enjoyable parts of sex and lovemaking. Both before and during sex, try to keep your thoughts on the pleasure of what happens/is happening. Concentrating on the positive rather than the negative may help to reduce the impact of the pain.

- Have you gone to a pain clinic where psychologists and other professionals specialize in pain management? You'll be taught how to reduce the effect of pain by the way you think and hold your body. It's definitely worth considering.
- If the problem is lack of lubrication, the solution is quite simple. Find something to substitute for your own wetness. Pharmacies sell special lubricants made for this purpose. Before beginning sex, spread some on your vulva and clitoris and, if you want to include penetration in your sexual activity, inside your vagina and on the penis/dildo/vibrator/fingers.

  Do this whether you're on your own or with a partner (it might be fun to have your partner do it for you). Don't be afraid to tell your partner when you need to use the lubricant. Every moment of delay is a moment of anxiety about pain, and, even one moment of anxiety can make your sexual arousal disappear quick as a flash.
- If you're having sex with a partner, *talk*. Don't suffer in silence. Talk about what's happening to you during sex. Talk about your avoidance of the pain. Talk about what kind of sex works best for you. Don't assume your partner can read your mind as to which activity or position or time is less painful for you. And don't forget, two heads are often better than one when it comes to creative ideas.

### Secondary pain

Let's now turn to secondary pain and what you can do about it. Firstly, you need to be convinced that there is no physical reason for pain to occur. If necessary, see your doctor to check on this. Are you the worrying type who finds it hard to believe there's no physical cause of your pain (even when you've seen the test results)?

If so, check it out yourself. First, have a relaxing bath or shower. In your bedroom or somewhere else that's private and comfortable, put some massage oil or lubricant on your fingers, and try *gently* stroking your vulva, clitoris, and vaginal entrance. This will show you that touching these areas doesn't feel painful. Keep stroking until you feel confident that pain isn't going to occur.

If you still feel worried, get some help from a psychologist or therapist. Find out why you worry in this way and what you can do about it. Then return to this page and continue with the Programs I suggest.

Once you know there is no infection or other condition that could cause pain, try saying the following positive statements to yourself.

## positive statements to overcome the fear of pain

- I can now let myself go sexually. I have no medical condition that will give me pain.
- As long as I relax and enjoy my sexual pleasure, there's nothing to give me pain.

Repeat these statements, listening carefully to the words. Don't worry if it's hard to fully believe what you're saying. Nothing changes in an instant. However, these positive statements can stop you from automatically reacting with anxiety and tension during sex. Here's how:

- Twice each day for the next two weeks, repeat the statements out loud. I suggest once in the morning before you get out of bed and once at night before you go to sleep.
- Before you begin any sexual activity say them again, out loud. Remember to breathe deeply and relax as you say them.
- During sex, if you find yourself becoming tense and anxious, repeat your positive statements. If you're with a partner, tell him or her to stop for a moment. Then breathe deeply and say them to yourself or out loud. Wait until you feel relaxed before you continue with sex.

If you're having difficulty doing this, you may need to relearn how to relax and to become aroused without anxiety. The Personal Change Program and Couple Change Program can be very helpful in doing this. Try the Personal Change Program first, perhaps skipping over the first two steps if they seem too simple. If you find you're able to orgasm without difficulty, move to the Couple Change Program (but follow it exactly as I've described).

If you're still having difficulty, let a therapist help you find out where the problem lies.

## use of medications |

IF YOU'RE TAKING medications or drugs, it's very important that you know exactly how these may affect your level of sexual arousal. Ask your doctor. If he or she doesn't seem to know, go to someone else. Don't be embarrassed to find out. You *need* this information and, unfortunately, too many doctors don't provide it (maybe *they're* embarrassed!).

If the medication could be making it difficult for you to orgasm at this time, check with your doctor as to whether lowering the dose or changing to another brand would help.

If it's antidepressant medication that you're taking, either for depression or anxiety, therapy with an experienced psychologist may help you to replace your medication with psychological techniques (or at least allow you to be on a lower dose).

What do you do if your medications can't be changed? Then there's no point being angry or upset because you can't orgasm. These emotions will keep you so focused on the negative side of sex (what you're missing out on) that you'll ignore any positive aspects of the situation.

Try to put your attention on the enjoyment you do feel, both from your body and the sexual situation. Orgasm is, after all, only one part of the whole sexual picture.

Have you made "having an orgasm" the only goal of sex? Have you become fixed on having an orgasm—*just because you can't?* Check this out.

Take some time to think about all the nice things that come from being sexual. Remind yourself that orgasm is simply *one* of these. Remember that your arousal hill has scenery that can be most enjoyable.

You may have to talk to your partner about this new focus on the positive rather than the negative. He or she may have picked up your frustration over not having an orgasm, and may have felt helpless at being unable to do something to make you happier. Talk the situation through, until you both come to the same idea: that it's the fun, closeness and pleasure of your sexual relationship that are important, rather than orgasms.

Keep in mind, though, that frustration and disappointment (negative feelings) can dampen your sexual feelings. So your difficulty with orgasm may be a combination of the medication *and* your negative approach. If you think this might be happening, turn to chapters 13 and 14. The Programs I outline can help you to feel as sexually aroused as possible. As you complete them, don't be surprised if you find your level of sexual pleasure increasing, even if you're still unable to have an orgasm because of the medication you're taking.

## dealing with changes in health |

YOU MAY BE experiencing difficulty with orgasm because of the effects of disease, injury, physical changes, or mental health changes. This can be upsetting and frustrating. To add to your problems, you may get little or no information from your doctors about the effects of these conditions on your sexual arousal. As I mentioned earlier, the medical profession can feel just as awkward about sexuality as the rest of the population. So, any questions you ask may be met with silence or superficial answers.

However, you need to know! Don't be afraid to ask. And keep asking until you completely understand. If your doctor can't give you the information, ask for a referral to one who can. Here are some questions you should ask:

- What effect will this condition/injury/disease/surgery have on my sexual feelings in the short term? In the long term?
- Will it affect my ability to get aroused? To orgasm? Will it change the way I experience an orgasm?
- Are there medications, drugs or other treatments that can help me to feel (more) sexual?

You should also try to check whether the information you're getting is up-to-date.

If you find that your difficulty with orgasm is temporary, you may have to learn to accept the situation as it is, until your health recovers. Stay positive in your thinking and remind yourself that orgasm is only one part of sexuality. Check whether different kinds of stroking to your clitoris will help. You may need a firmer, or longer, touch. Also check whether there are any medications that can help to reduce uncomfortable symptoms (such as genital soreness or sensitivity, spasms, and joint pain).

However, if the situation is not going to change, there are several things you can do to increase your enjoyment of sex and possibly strengthen sexual arousal. Are you prepared to change the way you get aroused? Are you open to learning new sexual triggers? If you are, then try the following suggestions:

- Learn to focus on the enjoyable parts of sex. See the previous section under Use of Medications where I talked about how to do this. It's a rare woman who feels absolutely nothing sexually because of a physical condition. Take some time, therefore, to learn about what is and isn't possible for you sexually. If you're able, explore your body when alone.
  - Are there positions that are more arousing than others?
  - Are there positions that are easier to get into?
  - Is there a time of the day when you're more likely to feel turned on?
  - Are there some ways of being touched that are more arousing than others? Try using a vibrator or dildo. Perhaps you now need a harder, or longer, touch to arouse you. Using a vibrator or dildo may make this easier.
  - Has *where* you like to be touched also changed?
- Explore your body to see if *other* parts have become more sensitive to sexual pleasure. This often happens if our vulva and clitoris become less able to respond with sexual sensations.

- And what about your fantasies? Do you need to make them more intense, more exotic?
- Can you use memories of previous sexual times to fill in the gaps you now have in your arousal? When it seems to get to a certain level and doesn't go any further, try fantasizing that you're having an orgasm. Make your memories of orgasm part of your fantasies. Remember, sexual arousal is as much a psychological reaction as a physical one. So, even with a physical condition that makes orgasm difficult, it may be possible to experience the feeling of orgasm with the help of our memories.
- The setting can also play a part in helping you to understand your sexual potential. Many women with health problems need to focus on being comfortable during sex. Of course, this is very important. But they often forget to *also* make the setting romantic and intimate, which means it will be harder to get into a sexual mood. Women with mental health problems also need to be in a setting that will help them to relax and focus on the enjoyable side of life. Play nice music, dim the lights or use candles—even if you're on your own. This will help you to focus more on your sexuality and less on your physical or mental condition.
- If necessary, see your doctor for medications that may help to relieve pain, burning sensations, dryness, fatigue, stiffness, spasms, bladder/bowel problems and so on.

When you've explored your sexuality on your own, try doing the same with your partner. Don't forget to find out which of the five senses (sight, sound, smell, touch, taste) seems to give you the most sexual pleasure.

---

Well, that sounds better than what I've been doing. I just gave up after my accident. Thought because the feelings were different I might as well forget sex.

---

You're not the only woman I've heard say this, believe me. I try to encourage everyone not to "give up." Yes, sometimes sexual feelings *do* change. That's why you have to explore yourself and find out what you can now feel and do. You need to find out how you react sexually *now*, without comparing yourself to how you *were*. Most importantly, you need to learn how to enjoy who you are now.

Remember, the only person who can become the expert on your sexuality is *you*. No one else can do it. It's up to you to take the time to discover your sexual potential. If you're worried about how far your physical condition will let you go with this, check with a doctor who is an expert in these matters.

There's an interesting story told by the sexology researcher, Dr. Beverly Whipple, which emphasizes the need for women to become the experts on their own sexuality. She noted that paraplegic women often said they felt orgasms, even when they had little or no sensation in their vulva and clitoris, due to spinal nerve damage. However, many medical practitioners dismissed these claims of orgasm because it was commonly assumed that paraplegic women could not get aroused or feel a climax.

After doing careful research, Dr. Whipple found that these women were *right* about themselves. She and her research team found that when paraplegic women were stimulated in the vagina with a vibrator, they did in fact experience an orgasm. The feelings of sexual arousal were sent to the brain by a different nerve (the vagus nerve) than that used by nonparaplegic women (the spinal cord). If the women studied had not become experts on their own sexuality, Dr. Whipple's research might never have been done.

If you have a spinal cord injury, therefore, you might like to check out whether you can feel sexual pleasure by using a vibrator inside your vagina. Don't forget to explore the rest of your body at the same time. You'll probably find that some new areas have become more sensitive and, if touched, may now turn you on sexually. And don't forget that you can still trigger sexual interest by your thoughts and senses, as do women without spinal cord injury.

❧

OF COURSE, NO matter what your physical or mental condition is, all the exploring in the world won't help if you're quite negative about your health. Many women feel angry, frustrated, upset, left out, bitter, and withdrawn about the changes to their health. These reactions are *very* understandable.

However, it's probably not wise to try to change the way you experience your sexual pleasure while you're feeling this way. Your negativity will only make you tense and distant from your partner. And, you *know* what that will do to your sexual arousal! There's no harm in waiting until you're in a better frame of mind. If you find it difficult to make an adjustment to the changes in your health, get some professional help. You may be surprised how useful this can be.

Of course, feeling positive won't do you much good if you have a partner who is frightened, concerned or just plain negative about your medical condition. If this is the case, the *two* of you would benefit from professional help.

It's important to take a positive approach to all aspects of your health. Being healthy covers eating well, getting enough sleep, keeping up muscle tone where you can, drinking in moderation, not smoking, and so on. I'm sure you know all this. But, don't forget to put regular sex on your list of "what I should do to stay healthy." It is just as important to keep the blood flowing into the pelvic area as to other parts of your body. So is taking time to enjoy yourself.

The Personal Change and Couple Change Programs outlined in the next two chapters help women to explore their sexuality. I would suggest you read through these Programs and use them as part of your own attempts to understand your sexual potential. You may have to adapt some parts (e.g., positions) to fit your own needs. For example, you may be unable to touch your own body or genitals without using some object such as a vibrator tied to a handle. However, the main guidelines should still be helpful to your explorations.

Another line of help for women with physical and medical conditions is the use of medications, nutritional supplements, hormones, and devices that aim to improve sexual arousal and orgasm.

Now, before you go rushing off to your doctor for a magic pill, let me warn you that, at this time, many medications and supplements are still being tested, and the long-term effects may be unknown. Some can have unpleasant side effects, such as nausea or extreme clitoral sensitivity. What is more, some women don't get the benefits from particular drugs and devices that others do—which can be most disappointing. As if this weren't enough, some drugs and devices aren't approved for use in certain countries, and they won't be until more testing has been done.

I've described some of the **medications, supplements, hormones**, and **devices** below, but you should also discuss the use of these with a doctor who knows about their effects on sexuality.

## MEDICATIONS
### Viagra (sildenafil)

Viagra, now well known to many people, allows the clitoris to become physically aroused by working on chemicals that open up the blood vessels. This lets the blood flow more easily into the erectile tissue of the clitoris. In chapter 3 you learned that increased blood flow makes the clitoris more sensitive, increases vaginal lubrication and helps to build sexual arousal to a level where orgasm can occur.

Viagra and similar drugs are no longer seen as the wonder cure for women's orgasm problems, as they were once promoted, with results being positive for some women and not for others. It would seem that women with conditions as different as spinal cord injury, nerve damage due to surgery, menopause, multiple sclerosis, and negative reactions to antidepressants may have their level of arousal and ability to have an orgasm improved by Viagra.

Keep in mind, though, that some women with a physical condition may be helped, while others with the same condition may not. And, interestingly, when studies of Viagra are carried out, many women who are given a pill that looks like Viagra, but is not (called a placebo), also show improvement in arousal and orgasm. This reminds us that there's more to arousal and orgasm than physical changes: paying more attention to your sexual reactions; holding a positive attitude towards sexuality; the "right" touch to your clitoris and body; and being open to things that trigger your sexual excitement are just as important. All these ingredients combine to make the orgasm "cake." Viagra may be able to help blood flow to the clitoris in some women, but it can't "invent" the willingness to feel sexual or make your partner sexually exciting.

### Other medications

For women who take medications that stop them from having an orgasm, there may be help from *other* medications that can overcome these effects. Check with an experienced doctor about whether you are able to take these drugs; not all women are.

Check, too, whether there are newer drugs available for your particular medical condition that have less effect on sexuality. The antidepressant bupropion, for example, is supposed to actually improve the likelihood of having orgasm. Bupropion has been found to have positive, not negative, effects on arousal and orgasm. While tests are still continuing, it seems that this medication can help women to have an orgasm and improve its strength, too.[15]

### Creams or lotions

These products are rubbed on the clitoris and vulva. Their manufacturers claim that they increase clitoris sensitivity and blood flow to the clitoris, and so increase the chance of orgasm. They're often promoted in magazines and by telephone marketing.

*Be careful.* Some of these creams are promoted as being the answer to *every* woman's *every* sexual problem. But there are so many different reasons for women's sexual difficulties that it's unlikely any one approach will be *the* answer.

What are these creams made of? Good question. Sometimes it's impossible to know. The ingredients aren't written on the container or in the brochures. Nor are possible side effects. And, most haven't been around long enough to see if there are any long-term effects.

Where information is available, ingredients common to most creams are L-Arginine (which is available from health stores) and menthol. L-Arginine is believed to play a minor part in the chemical reactions that help the clitoris to become aroused. Menthol tends to give a tingly feeling when rubbed onto the skin. That will certainly make you pay attention to your clitoris, won't it?

Be sensible and don't use anything without checking what it is. Ask your doctor before using any cream. Get all the information about how it works. Find out if there's any information on side effects and long-term use. Then make a decision about whether it can help you or not.

## NUTRITIONAL SUPPLEMENTS

The better your health, the more likely you are to be interested in sex and able to respond physically, mentally, and emotionally in a positive way to sexual triggers. Some nutritional products may be able to help you feel in better health.

One study found that a product that included the supplements L-Arginine, vitamins, minerals, ginseng, ginkgo, and damiana led to improvement in clitoral sensitivity and more frequent orgasm.[16]

## HORMONES

Use of hormones can sometimes help to overcome the effects of aging, menopause and some medical conditions. Keep in mind, however, that they're only one part of the answer to improving arousal. Hormones won't fix negative attitudes, destructive sexual habits, or a poor relationship.

### Estrogen

Low levels of estrogen can lead to mood swings, vaginal dryness and a thinning of the genital skin tissue. Although none of these has to lead to orgasm difficulties, they can make you less able to enjoy sex. This loss of enjoyment may then stop you from getting aroused enough to orgasm.

Using estrogen supplements (hormone replacement therapy) can overcome these physical changes and help you feel in the mood for sex. However, research suggests that some forms of estrogen replacement should only be used for short periods of time or, in some women, not at all. Talk to your doctor about the types of estrogen that are available and decide which is best suited to you.

### Androgens

*Testosterone*. The hormone testosterone is produced in a woman's ovaries, just like estrogen. It is often thought that a low level of one type of testosterone, known as *free testosterone*, is responsible for low interest in sex for women. There is actually poor evidence for this, but low testosterone levels may effect a woman's interest indirectly—for example by reducing her ability to respond to sexual triggers.

What has this got to do with having orgasms, you ask? Good question. There are links between the two areas, of course. You won't get aroused if you're not interested, and if you're not aroused, you won't orgasm. But, as I mentioned in chapter 1, the physical *and* psychological causes of lack of sexual interest can be quite different from those for arousal and orgasm difficulties.

Unfortunately, some medical practitioners lump all women's sexual difficulties together. As a result, women with orgasm difficulties are sometimes given medications or hormones (such as testosterone) on the (wrong) assumption that increasing sexual *interest* will lead to orgasms. Can you imagine how upsetting it is to find that the instant orgasm you were expecting doesn't happen?

However, testosterone, especially in the form of creams, is also used to strengthen skin tissue in the vulva and clitoris. This can then improve the flow of blood to the area and, in some women, increase clitoral sensation. As you will remember, good blood flow to the erectile tissues of the clitoris is one important step in overcoming orgasm difficulties. So, testosterone creams may play a part in helping women with physical and medical conditions to increase sensitivity and feelings of sexual pleasure. These changes may then lead to orgasm.

Testosterone is not suitable for everyone. If the dose is too high it can have unwelcome side effects, such as acne, extra body hair and low voice. Always check with your doctor before using any form of testosterone, and make sure the level of testosterone in your body is carefully monitored. Find out about its suitability for you, possible benefits and side effects (including long-term effects).

*DHEA (Dehydroepiandrosterone).* This is another androgen-type hormone that is present in women's bodies, and like other hormones, decreases in amount with aging. It converts to forms of estrogen and testosterone and, among other things, plays a significant part in skin sensation and touch. It's thought that low levels of DHEA may contribute to loss of clitoral sensitivity and well-being, as well as increasing fatigue. Some menopausal women report that taking DHEA seems to make their level of arousal stronger, their clitoris more sensitive, and their orgasms more intense. However, like other hormones, there's still a lot we don't know about the immediate or long-term effects of DHEA. And it isn't available in all countries.

## DEVICES

There are several *devices* (also known as sex toys) that can help with sexual arousal and orgasm. Some, like vibrators, provide a strong rhythmic movement that may help women with low nerve and muscle sensitivity. Others fit over the clitoris like a cap and gently suck it, stimulating the flow of blood to this area.

These devices work on increasing your levels of arousal so that orgasm will happen more easily. They are usually battery-operated, but there is some experimentation with one that is surgically connected to the nerves of the spinal cord and, by use of a remote control, is intended to trigger physical reactions that may lead to orgasm.

Like drugs, some devices may be useful to you, others may not. And some will be available where you live, whereas others won't have been approved (yet?). If you decide to use a device, take the time to find out whom the device is intended to help and how it works.

---

That's all very well, but an orgasm is a bit more than nerves and blood flow. You said it yourself. I don't want sex to be all about a piece of machinery or pills.

---

I can understand that. We all know that sex for women is more than just orgasms. It's about what we feel, what we think, the mood we're in, how romantic the setting is, and so on. Our psychological reactions are as important as our physical ones, if not *more* important.

I can understand how talking about medications, devices, and so on will seem to focus too much on getting you to "have an orgasm," rather than on enjoying your feelings of sexual pleasure. If you feel uncomfortable with this approach, you can do one of two things:

1. **Stop worrying about having orgasms.**

   Concentrate on enjoying the feelings of sexual pleasure you do get: being touched, the closeness with a partner and so on. Enjoy all this to the full, and take the pressure off yourself to orgasm. Think positively about what you have sexually, rather than what you don't have.

2. **Change the way you think about taking medications, supplements or hormones, or using devices.**

   We all have a set of conditions that help us to get turned on. All you have to do is add one more thing to your list— medications, devices, and so on. Look at them as simply another trigger that you need to become sexually turned on. And keep in mind, we're only talking about *one* item on your list. There are still many other things you need to get aroused.

☙

I CAN'T FINISH this section without mentioning that, when available, medications are sometimes used by women who are physically healthy. This can be a serious problem if the causes of your orgasm difficulties are ignored or given brief attention. For example, swallowing any number of pills won't make it easier to orgasm if the problem is your lack of attraction to your partner.

On the other hand, in some circumstances, medications *may* be helpful if used with psychological and sexual therapy. For example, if, as a result of relationship, personal, or other factors, you've completely lost confidence in your ability to orgasm, the use of medications or creams might help (so, too, might a vibrator). If you feel stronger sensations in your clitoris, your confidence may return. This can then encourage you to make the personal, sexual, or relationship changes you *know* have to be made.

Keep in mind, however, that while medications and devices may shorten the time you're in psychological and sexual therapy, they can't replace the changes you need to make.

# 13

# learning to orgasm in private
## your personal change program

IN THIS CHAPTER I'm going to teach you to orgasm on your own. Then, in the next chapter I'll describe the Couple Change Program for those who want to orgasm with a partner. Actually, these Programs teach much more than how to orgasm, so be prepared to find them enjoyable as well as helpful.

## the advantages of the personal change program

I MENTIONED PREVIOUSLY that learning to orgasm is often easier when practiced alone. There are real advantages to being on your own. All you have to do is concentrate on *you*.

- There's no worrying about what your partner's thinking or feeling.

- You're able to go at your own pace, without feeling pressure from a partner.
- You can learn to relax and enjoy your sexual passion without embarrassment.
- You can learn about your arousal patterns without interruption.
- You're free to explore new things because you're in control of what you do and think.

I *strongly* recommend you do the Personal Change Program, *whether you're in a relationship or not*. Not only is it an easier way for you to learn to climax, it's also an important first step to being able to orgasm with a partner.

---

But aren't you really talking about masturbation? As
a child I learned "nice" women don't do that.

---

You're right that I will be teaching you how to masturbate. This simply means learning to touch yourself on the body and genitals in a way that will allow you to become sexually aroused. It's one way of feeling sexual pleasure and is enjoyed by many women.

Actually, women often masturbate without realizing what they're doing. For example, they squeeze their legs together, rock gently while holding something between their legs or push against an object such as a bike seat. All these activities can give pleasure because the clitoris is touched and pressed.

However, I realize some women find it difficult to think about becoming aroused by touching their own body. They've been taught by parents, religious organizations, or the larger community that women shouldn't do this.

There are also myths about masturbation that sometimes scare women away from trying it. Most of these myths are just plain silly and wrong. Did you hear the one that says, "Women who mastur-bate will become sexually promiscuous"? What nonsense!

Unfortunately, some women think that sex with a partner is the only "real" way of enjoying their sexual feelings. To them, masturbation is a second-best way, something you do when you're on your own. I see this idea as just another myth, created, perhaps, to keep women from enjoying their own sexual pleasure.

Neither masturbation nor sex with a partner is better or worse than the other. They're simply *different* ways in which to express ourselves sexually.

**The truth is, many, many women DO masturbate, and enjoy it very much.**

Interestingly, *most* men masturbate. They don't seem to feel worried or guilty about masturbating. This isn't surprising. It's *women*, not men, who are usually given negative messages about masturbation and discouraged from enjoying their sexuality.

By the way, don't think it's only single women who masturbate. Many women in satisfying relationships also enjoy being sexual in this way. They see masturbation as a different way of feeling sexual and just as enjoyable as having sex with their partner.

I hope you're able to learn to become highly aroused and to orgasm during masturbation.

**It's often the best way to understand how your own body becomes sexually aroused**

AND

**women who can orgasm on their own usually find it easier to orgasm with a partner**

AND

**women who masturbate are more likely to orgasm than women who don't.**

Look at the figures found in one study:[17]

---

**Women who masturbated once a week or more:**
- 81% usually or always had an orgasm
- 19% sometimes/never had an orgasm

**Women who masturbated one to six times a year:**
- 67% usually or always had an orgasm
- 3% sometimes/never had an orgasm

It's clear, isn't it? Most women who masturbate are likely to orgasm. That's why I'm so keen for you to try the Personal Change Program. Shortly I'll outline the Program in detail so you can get started.

If you can already orgasm when masturbating, *but it seems like hard work*, I recommend you also read through this chapter to learn how to become highly aroused more easily. Remember, orgasms don't have to be hard work. So, give yourself the chance to learn how to enjoy your sexual pleasure more easily.

If you enjoy masturbating, but can't orgasm, you may be able to skip over Steps 1 and 2 of the Program. Read through them first and decide for yourself. *Don't* skip the other steps, however, even if you're tempted.

# concerns about doing the personal change program

I'M SURE SOME of you are still wondering whether to try the Program. If you have any concerns, take a moment to stop and think about what it is that worries you.

## WOMEN WHO FEEL RELUCTANT TO MASTURBATE

You may be like many women who find it difficult to put their reluctance to masturbate into words. Perhaps you feel a vague negativity about it, a carryover from childhood, when you were taught that girls shouldn't be too free with their sexuality. Perhaps you saw someone masturbating as a child and from this developed a negative feeling about it.

Take some time to think about where you learned your negative attitudes and reactions towards masturbation. Write these in the space below. Then write down where you learned to think this way.

## my attitudes towards masturbation

**What I think and feel about masturbation:**

_____

_____

**Where I learned these attitudes and feelings:**

_____

_____

Now, ask yourself whether the things you *think and feel about masturbation* are really your beliefs or the ideas of the people you grew up with. Sometimes we hold beliefs simply because they were taught to us as a child.

You may be holding on to attitudes that don't fit how you think as an adult. The problem is, while you carry negative ideas about masturbation around in your head, it's hard to take a positive approach to it. Take some time, therefore, to think about your childhood lessons on masturbation. You may be surprised to find you no longer agree with them.

---

Can there be anything positive about masturbation?
Isn't it just being selfish?

---

No, I don't see masturbation as being selfish. For the time you're actually touching yourself and enjoying sexual feelings, you will indeed be focused on your feelings. But it would be the same if you were listening to music or taking time to read a magazine.

Sometimes it's important to take time for yourself. This certainly doesn't mean you'll *never* have time for others. For example, if an emergency arose while you were masturbating, I'm sure, like most women, you'd stop what you were doing and rush to help. That's hardly selfish, is it?

And to answer your first question, masturbation can have some *very* positive effects. It can:

- make us experts on our own sexual arousal
- make us feel worthwhile (for example, because we've made the decision to do something for ourselves rather than blindly follow someone else's attitudes)
- improve our self-confidence in sexual areas
- free us up from having to wait for our partner to be in a sexual mood
- free us up from having to *have* a partner
- relax us and provide a way of relieving stress (believe me, an orgasm is as good as a relaxing bath—and better than sedatives!)
- leave nice memories to think over during the day
- offer the chance to learn *new* ways of becoming aroused

So let me encourage you to think about how masturbation can add to your life. And, if possible, *try* the Program. Don't say no just because it was the first word that came into your head. Think through my comments. See if you can allow yourself to do what countless women happily do on a regular basis.

## WOMEN WHO ARE STRONGLY AGAINST MASTURBATION

If you feel most strongly that the Personal Change Program is not for you because of religious or other reasons, then go directly to the Couple Change Program. If you don't have a partner at the moment, use the time to concentrate on any other areas of change you need to make.

However, I'd like to urge you *not* to stop reading this chapter on the Personal Change Program. I'd be surprised if there weren't a tidbit or two of information for you to think over.

# a bit of planning before we begin ... |

LIKE ANY NEW project, it's important to do a bit of planning before you get started.

1. **Make sure you have some private (and preferably quiet) space to do the exercises.**

   If you live with a partner, you'll need to talk with him or her about having a room to yourself for the exercises. Make sure you won't be interrupted by outside noise (for example, your children banging on the door!). Your attention needs to be on *you*, without worrying what's happening outside.

   To put your mind at ease, you may want to lock the door or wait until there's no one else at home. There's no point starting anything if you're going to constantly worry that someone could walk into the room. If you have children, the lock may allow you to do the Program without fear of being interrupted.

   ------

   Oh dear, I don't think I can do this. . . . I'm so used
   to being there whenever I'm needed.

   ------

I know, I know! It's hard taking time at home just for you and can feel strange shutting a partner or children out of the bedroom. Like you, many women feel guilty about this.

Try telling yourself . . .

- They'll survive without me.
- My partner is perfectly capable of coping for half an hour.
- I'm entitled to some time for myself.
- Learning how to orgasm will make me a happier person and then everyone will benefit.

In fact, tell yourself anything that will allow you to do the exercises without punishing yourself with GUILT.

## 2. Plan in advance when you're going to do the exercises.

If you don't, the week will flash by without a single moment devoted to your sexuality. So open your diary and on three days write in, *Personal Change Program—ten to twenty minutes*. Yes, that's all you need, ten minutes (three times a week) at first, building up to twenty minutes on three occasions. Three times a week is necessary to give you steady progress. Obviously, the less you do it, the longer it will take for changes to occur.

By the way, *don't* plan an appointment for immediately after the exercise. Otherwise, you'll be looking at the clock and won't be able to relax.

Try to avoid doing the exercise when you're too tired; it will seem like a real effort and you'll start in a negative frame of mind.

One more thing, if possible, make sure the room you'll be doing your exercise in has been warmed or cooled beforehand. It won't be much fun if you're freezing cold or bathed in perspiration.

## 3. Go shopping. Find some gentle music to play while you're doing the exercise.

Try to choose something without words (otherwise you might start singing along and forget to do the exercise). Buy some candles to make the setting more romantic. This will help you get into a positive mood. You'll also need some massage oil to rub over your skin, so your fingers can glide more easily. Remember, this is going to be a nice time for *you*.

## 4. If you can get the time, take a bath or shower before beginning.

And while you do this, there's nothing to stop you having a few sexual fantasies. Imagine a romantic or sexy story, picture a sexy scene with someone who turns you on (or *imagine* someone who turns you on). Let your mind wander over whatever seems to raise a spark of sexual interest.

Play your music while in the bath or shower, and continue playing it while doing the exercises. Light the candles or dim the lights. By the time you begin your exercise, you should be feeling relaxed and ready to start. If not, spend a few moments lying quietly and breathing deeply.

### 5. Don't pressure yourself with expectations of what should happen.

I know there's going to be a certain amount of pressure in just trying to follow the first two points outlined above. So, it's really important that you don't add to it by placing demands on yourself to get turned on or reach orgasm.

*I don't expect anything*, other than that you follow the Program as closely as possible and see what happens. Provided nothing distracts you from this or causes you to lose motivation, you'll do fine.

Relax, then, and don't try to rush ahead of me or yourself. Give yourself the time to change those old habits I talked about in earlier chapters. This can't be done overnight, so don't try to speed up the Program. There's no prize for working through the Program in the shortest time possible.

### 6. Learn to use your fingers rather than rely on a vibrator.

If you've found in the past that a vibrator is the best way for you to get aroused, it may seem a bit daunting to think about doing the Program using your fingers.

Now, there's nothing wrong with using a vibrator to arouse yourself. In fact, for women with certain disabilities (for example, women with arthritis in their hands) this is an ideal way (and may be the only way) to complete the Program.

However, if you have no disabilities and this is the *only* way you can get turned on, then I believe it's important that you learn to use fingers just as easily. That way, you have a choice. So, for the moment, leave the vibrator on the cabinet next to you. I may suggest you use it at different times during the Program.

### 7. Be realistic and positive.

Change, as I said earlier, takes time. Your body and mind need time to learn new patterns of reacting, thinking and feeling. The Program may take weeks or months to complete. To keep yourself moving forward, remind yourself why you're doing it:

---

- I'm learning to be an expert on my own arousal.
- I'm learning how to let myself be more highly aroused.
- I need to give myself enough time to learn new ways of becoming aroused.
- It's a good way of learning to orgasm.

---

And try to be realistic. For example, there's absolutely no point in telling yourself an orgasm will happen next week. Dear reader, I'm not a miracle worker!

Find something positive to say about having orgasms that is also realistic. For example:

> *Now that I understand the causes of my orgasm difficulties, there's nothing to stop me learning to become highly aroused and to orgasm.*

That's believable and achievable, don't you think?

---

Hmm. . . . Still, it's hard not to feel impatient.
I'm probably the only one of my friends
who can't orgasm.

---

Maybe, maybe not, but what's a few more months. . . ?

### 8. Being a little uncomfortable is fine.

I've broken the Program into easy steps and, hopefully, you'll be able to move from step to step without too much trouble.

Don't worry if at first you feel anxious about what you're being asked to do. Perhaps you're a bit nervous because it's something new. Or maybe those old negative beliefs or memories about masturbation are affecting you.

It will help if you keep in mind that most women become more comfortable as time goes by. I'll usually suggest you do an exercise on three occasions within a week. There's a good reason for this. On the first occasion, you may feel a bit anxious. On the second, you'll become a little more comfortable. And on the third, you could even begin to feel relaxed.

The more you practise each exercise, the easier it will be to do and the more at ease you'll feel. So be prepared to try each step of the Program, even if you feel a bit anxious at different times. You'll be surprised at how soon you become comfortable.

### 9. If possible, tell your partner what you're doing.

As you work your way through each exercise, talk to your partner about what you're doing and how you're feeling. Don't worry if you feel a bit embarrassed. The more you talk, the easier it will become.

Believe me, it's much easier to let your partner know what's happening. He or she can take the kids away from the house for a while or, in some other way, help you to get the privacy you need.

Partners are often more sympathetic and encouraging when they see that you're keen to learn how to orgasm. They can also become more understanding of the difficulty you have from hearing about the exercise and how you're going with it.

By the way, tell your partner in advance that he or she

doesn't have to solve any problems or offer advice unless you ask for it. All you need is a friendly ear and the occasional (or regular) hug.

### 10. Be creative.

If you have some physical condition that makes it difficult for you to move, touch, or lay flat, take some time to adapt the exercise. You need to be comfortable. This is your chance to be creative (but stick to the Program as much as possible).

Try sitting in a chair or raising your head with pillows if this feels more comfortable. You may need to tie a vibrator to a long handle. Remember to use this at low speed if you have a condition that leads to muscle spasms or if you tend to go numb around the clitoris and vulva.

Try to do the Program at a time of the day that is less painful or stressful for you.

Make sure you use massage oil or lubrication so that you're not rubbing on dry skin (which can be painful).

## the personal change program |

BEFORE YOU BEGIN the Program, I want to make a suggestion. Read one step, *then do it before reading about the next step*. When you've completed the step you're on, *then* go on to the next step. Otherwise, you may look at the last step, panic because you don't think you can do it, and give up.

If you follow the Program in this way, you'll become quite confident of your ability to get sexually aroused. By the time you get to the last step, you should feel ready to try it (without any sign of panic).

Because you're unlikely to be ready for it *right now*, don't make things difficult for yourself by jumping steps. Each step follows on from the other. There's nothing to be gained from starting in the middle of the Program.

Let's begin.

## STEP 1: exploring

Find a time when you'll have no interruptions for about ten minutes. Begin by lying naked on a comfortable bed or lounge. If you're really uncomfortable with being naked, wear a loose top. Place your arms beside you and let your legs fall open.

Shut your eyes and see if you can simply *notice*, or be *aware* of each part of your body in turn. Start from your head and work down. *Feel* your head. *Feel* your neck. Feel your shoulders—and so on, right down to your toes. Take your time. If you rush, you'll only be *thinking about* what you're doing—which is not the same as being *aware*.

Check your breathing. It should be nice and easy—relaxed. Let your chest and stomach rise and fall with each breath. Check if there are any areas where you're tense. Wriggle your arms, legs, and pelvis to see how relaxed they are.

If you're feeling a little awkward or self-conscious, remember there's no one to judge you except yourself. And you've probably done enough of that.

Now, put your attention on your vulva and clitoris. Notice how these areas fit into the rest of your body. With your fingers, feel where they meet each leg. Feel the way they rest next to your buttocks. Stroke where your pubic hair meets your stomach.

Take a nice, easy breath and imagine the air flowing all the way down from your mouth, through your stomach, into your vulva and clitoris and down your legs.

❧

NEXT, LET'S EXPLORE your vulva and clitoris a little more. It's important to know how these parts of *you* look and feel. Many women have never looked at themselves—or have done so briefly and without much interest. Some only touch their outer genitals when washing (and then only with a cloth or soap).

Yet, our vulva and clitoris are part of our body, and we need to be as familiar with them as we are with our hands and face.

So, take a small hand mirror and, in a sitting or lying position, spend some time looking at your vulva and clitoris. Those with physical disabilities may need to attach the mirror to a rod for reach, or ask someone to hold it for them. Of course, this last suggestion means you're not alone, but you may prefer this to not being able to do the exercise at all.

While watching in the mirror, touch the different areas with your fingers: the outer labia or lips, the inner labia, the clitoris hood, the clitoris glans, the clitoris shaft (roll your finger backwards and forwards across the hood to find it lying just under the skin), the entrance to your vagina and finally, the area between the entrance to your vagina and your anus (the perineum). Use the illustration given earlier in this book to help you identify the areas. As you look and touch, say the name of each part of your genitals to yourself.

**Do this on two to three occasions in the next week** (until you feel quite comfortable looking at yourself and know exactly how you fit together). On one of these occasions, try drawing your genitals. Yes, I said *draw!* Now, now, I won't be asking you to hang your masterpiece in an art gallery. Just try it. The vulva and clitoris are cleverly put together, and you won't realize this fully until you try to draw them.

If you find at the end of the second or third occasion, there are *absolutely* no problems (you are relaxed and positive), move on to Step 2. If not, do Step 1 at least two more times and then check how you feel. If you've become fairly relaxed about what you're doing, move on to Step 2.

&#8788;

IF YOU FEEL uncomfortable looking at or touching the different parts of your genitals, check out why. Ask yourself, *What am I thinking about as I do this exercise?*

It's quite likely that you have been thinking negatively. See if you can identify what that negative thought might be. Think about where you learned this way of thinking. Ask yourself whether you still need to think this way. Remind yourself that negative thinking makes it hard to feel relaxed.

Women sometimes imagine that their outer genitals are ugly. For this reason they may feel uncomfortable about looking too closely. Try the next exercise to find out whether you see yourself as ugly or not. *Everyone* should try this exercise.

## my genitals are like a red, red . . . (?)

It has often been said that our vulva and outer clitoris are like a flower to look at.

Look at your genitals again in the mirror. See if you can choose a flower that reminds you of their shape. If you're having difficulty, wander around gardens (at another time, of course). Look through gardening books.

Don't pick any flower just because you like it. Every vulva/clitoris combination is different, and you should try to think of a flower that suits yours in particular.

Write the flower you've chosen below:

_____

It may surprise you, but I've heard at least a dozen different flowers named as reminding women of their genitals. One thing is certain. Once you find the flower that is like your vulva and clitoris, you won't be able to see them as ugly again.

If you're still having trouble feeling positive about this step of the Personal Change Program, remind yourself why you're doing it. I gave you some examples of positive thoughts earlier, but it doesn't hurt to repeat them here:

- This is the first step in learning to be an expert on my own arousal.
- This is the first step in learning how to let myself be more highly aroused, so I can feel an orgasm.

And remind yourself that:

- Many, many women look at their genitals from time to time; it's quite normal for me to do this.
- It's important to know my genitals as well as I know my own hand or face.
- I cannot hurt myself; I'm in control here.

Now, try the exercise again from the beginning. Try it again on another day. Do this until it can be carried out easily and without stress. Don't move to Step 2 until you're ready. There's no rush. You've waited this long, as I've said before, so another few months won't hurt.

If there's no change, get some help from a therapist who works in the sexuality area.

## STEP 2: EXPLORING SENSITIVITY

In this step you're going to learn a little more about your vulva, clitoris and vagina. You'll need to allow about fifteen minutes of private, uninterrupted time (you can take longer if you wish). Don't forget the candles and music, for they can help you get into a peaceful mood. You may want to use some talcum powder, massage oil, or lubricant on your fingers to help you stroke your body more easily. Nothing too scented, though. Otherwise, you'll soon be gasping for air, instead of gently relaxing.

Lie on the bed or a comfortable surface and shut your eyes. Take a few moments to notice all the parts of your body. Be aware of those areas where you feel tense. Breathe nice and easily, noticing your chest and stomach rising and falling.

Now, for a few moments, *stroke* all those parts of your body that you can reach. Try different types of stroking: hard, soft; quick, slow; pressing, sliding; whole hand, fingers. Notice how each of these movements makes you feel. Don't analyze. Don't judge your body. Try to stay focused on the pleasant feelings you get as you stroke your skin.

Next, I want you to stroke the different parts of your vulva and clitoris to see how sensitive they are to your touch. Some will be very sensitive and give you a nice feeling. Other areas may be less sensitive (but may still give a very nice feeling). There are no right or wrong ways to do this. Just stroke in a way that feels nice and *be aware* of what sensations you get as a result.

Try stroking in different directions and with different types of movements. However, remember, your clitoris is a *delicate* part of your body. A heavy hand will only distract you and make it difficult to detect levels of sensitivity. Be careful, too, when stroking directly on the glans or head of the clitoris because it can be VERY sensitive (don't say I didn't warn you).

It doesn't matter *what* sensations you get as you stroke. Don't think *about* them. Don't *judge* them. Don't try to figure out if they're sexual sensations or not. This isn't important. Just feel. The point of this exercise is to

**. . . see if you can identify which areas of your vulva and clitoris are more sensitive than others.**

That's all you have to do.

Remember, every woman is unique. No two women react in the same way. So, it doesn't matter what you've read about the sensations other women feel in their genitals. That information won't tell you much about *your* feelings. You need to find out about *your body*.

Explore! See what you can find out about your vulva and clitoris. Get to know your body. Your outer genitals, as I said earlier, are simply another part of your body. You should become familiar with how they react to touch, just as you're familiar with how your hands, shoulders or legs feel when touched.

As you explore yourself, try to identify which parts seem very sensitive, moderately sensitive, or of little sensitivity. Become familiar with the feelings you get when touching each part. Experiment with different kinds of touch and see if you get different reactions.

Move the labia and notice what effect this has on the clitoris. Do the same with the hood of skin covering the clitoris glans. See if you can feel the shaft of your clitoris and the branches (or legs) of the clitoris running under each labia towards your buttocks. Don't worry if you can't; they're not easy to detect and may be more obvious when you're sexually aroused. If you're feeling agile, try pulling your knees up towards your breasts and search for the clitoral legs this way (but it's not worth pulling a muscle over!).

See if you can tighten your lower pelvic muscles. Remember, these muscles play an important part in increasing sexual pleasure, so it's good to be aware of this part of your body. Imagine you're trying to pull your vagina up into your stomach. Tighten and let go several times. Notice if this has any effect on the feelings you get as you touch your clitoris. If you have difficulty finding these muscles, it may be because they're weak and need to be strengthened. If necessary, see a physiotherapist or other professional who specializes in helping women do this. You'll be given exercises to help build your muscle tone.

Now stroke around the entrance of your vagina. Slip your fingers into the entrance and stroke the skin. Notice how this feels. Try tightening the muscles around the vagina and see if this gives a different feeling. Move your fingers around so you can press the upper wall of your vagina (under the pubic bone). You may feel a spongy area: the G-spot. Don't worry if you can't:

- It's easier to feel when you're aroused.
- You may not be able to reach the area.
- If you're wearing a diaphragm for contraception, it may cover the G-spot.

Move to the perineum. It's a spongy area, similar to the G-spot, that can give a very pleasant feeling when touched. If you've been through childbirth, do your exploring gently. This area may have become extra sensitive as a result of a tearing of the skin when giving birth.

If you can reach, stroke and press the anus. You may be surprised at how sensitive this can be. Women who are paralyzed below the waist, or have had the nerves in their clitoris damaged, sometimes find that the anus remains very sensitive and pleasant to touch.

While doing this exercise, there are some (friendly) rules I want you to try and follow:

## rules for step 2

- **Let yourself enjoy this exercise**
  - Try not to hold back your enjoyment.
  - There's no reason to ration your feelings or to feel guilty about pleasant feelings.
- **Don't try too hard**
  - Remember, this is play, not work.

- **Don't pressure yourself with expectations**
  - Forget orgasms and wild sexual passion.
  - All you need to do is follow the exercise, learn to feel comfortable doing it, and remember to enjoy yourself along the way.

You may not feel much of anything at first. Especially if you don't usually notice how your body reacts. Stay relaxed, and eventually, you'll become aware of the sensations caused by your touch.

If you're having trouble feeling anything at all, and you've always used a vibrator in the past, it may be that you're having trouble adjusting to a softer, less regular touch. To help you to make the shift, do Step 2 several more times, using your fingers. Concentrate on the positive aspects of your new style of touching (e.g., the *softness* of your fingers).

If you have a physical condition that has reduced the sensitivity in your vulva and clitoris, try a firmer touch with your fingers or use a vibrator on low speed.

You can do this exercise lying down or half lying. It can be done with or without your hand mirror, but you should try it on some occasions without.

**Stroke and explore for about fifteen minutes on three occasions in the next week.** You'll soon become familiar with the amount of sensitivity that each area has for you. If you have physical difficulties or disabilities, you may need to either reduce or expand the time taken—and, if necessary, take two weeks for the exercise.

Once you can do Step 2 with ease and you're enjoying what you're doing, move on to Step 3. However, if you still feel a little uncomfortable after the third occasion, or have trouble keeping your attention on what you're doing, take another week or continue touching until you feel able to do the exercise more easily. But remember, if you're only doing the exercise once a week (or less), the positive effects will take a lot longer to show up.

Now, LET ME pause for a moment and chat to those of you who are feeling *very* uncomfortable with Step 2. Do you know why you feel this way? Is there a negative thought or two tucked away in your brain that is making you react? Here are examples of thoughts that women sometimes identify:

- *My mother would disown me if she knew I was doing this.*
- *It reminds me of when I was abused.*
- *Any moment now, this is going to give me pain.*

Remember, negative thoughts like these will lead you to tense up and switch off from your feelings. So go back and remind yourself of the positive reasons for doing this Program.

Remind yourself that you're doing it *for yourself*. Although others may have a different idea about how you should express (or *not* express) your sexuality, it's time to make up *your* mind about how sexual you want to be.

Keep yourself thinking about the present, not the past. Remind yourself that you are now an adult (or at least old enough to think for yourself).

Some women, who were forced to masturbate themselves or another person when they were younger, find they get confused between what they're doing *now* and what they did *then*. If this fits you, remind yourself that what you're doing in my Program is *quite different*. This exercise is for *your* pleasure and the whole situation is under your control. Remind yourself that it's okay to feel your own sexual pleasure. Whenever you get tense doing Step 2, say the following positive statement to yourself:

> This is not the past. Right now I'm
> safe and in control. It's time to relax
> and enjoy my feelings.

Some of you may be thinking and feeling negative because sex in the past has been associated with *pain* rather than pleasure. To help yourself become more comfortable, focus on what you're feeling *now*. If you no longer feel pain during sex, remind yourself of this. As you do the exercise I've outlined, check whether you're feeling pain. If not, tell yourself,

> There's no need to be tense. I'm not
> experiencing any pain now.

Of course, if you do feel pain, see your doctor immediately, and put the Program on hold until your pain is removed (or reduced as much as possible).

IF YOUR DISCOMFORT with Step 2 is based on feeling disinterested, take some time to identify *why* you feel this way. Check for negative thinking—this may give you a clue to what the problem is. For example, you may be thinking:

- *There are too many other things I should be doing.*
- *This isn't working, I hardly feel a thing.*

Both these examples are common for women who are so focused on *doing* things that when it comes time to relax and enjoy themselves, they find it difficult to do so.

If this fits you, then stay with the exercise; take that wonderful ability of yours to concentrate on *doing* things and *use* it to focus on what happens in your body when you touch your vulva and clitoris. Oh, and don't expect instant changes. We both know that isn't going to happen.

Whatever the reasons for feeling disinterested in the exercise, you'll need to decide what to do about them. You have two options. You can change the cause of your disinterest so the Program becomes attractive for you. If you need help to do this, put the Program on hold until you've seen a therapist and learn to become more motivated. But if you feel you can't or don't want to change the reasons for your disinterest, it may be better to leave the Program until a time when you're more positive about it.

The exception to all this would be feeling disinterested because you can already do the present exercise and you're bored. The simple answer is to move on to the next step.

## STEP 3: exploring pleasure

In this third step of the Personal Change Program, you continue to explore and learn. The exercise will take about fifteen minutes and should be done **six times over a two-week period.**

So, settle back onto a comfortable bed or other flat (and comfortable) surface and, as before, give yourself a few moments to relax and take notice of your body.

Now, focus on your pelvic area. If you can, bend your legs so that your knees are pointing upward while your feet remain on the bed. Try tensing and relaxing the muscles in the lower part of your stomach. Breathe in as you tighten, out as you relax. Do this several times. You'll probably feel the muscles in your buttocks and pelvis also tightening.

Next, press your lower back down toward the bed, then relax. Notice your hips rocking forward and back as you do this. Do it several times, taking note of how it also moves your vulva and clitoris. Be aware of the feelings you get in your vulva and clitoris from this movement. Try opening your legs wider to see if this makes a difference to the sensations you're feeling.

While keeping your attention on your pelvis, vulva, and clitoris, stroke your breasts, stomach, and any other areas that feel nice. Try to relax. If you can, imagine you're *melting* with the enjoyment of your touch. Enjoy your *sensuality.*

As you touch, try gently rocking your pelvis, just as you did before. Now, practice tightening the muscles around your clitoris and vagina. Remember to imagine pulling your vagina up into your stomach.

Then, when ready, begin to touch all those areas of your vulva, clitoris, vagina, and pelvic area that give you a pleasant feeling. You could think of this pleasant feeling as *sexual.* Don't forget to rub some massage or baby oil onto your fingers and genitals to help your fingers glide more easily over the skin.

Shut your eyes and focus on the feelings you get. Try to be *aware* and to *feel* the sensations. Don't think *about* (analyze) them; otherwise you'll start "spectatoring," or watching yourself in a judging way.

**The purpose of this exercise is to feel sensual and sexual pleasure.**

Allow yourself to feel and enjoy the sexual sensations *without pressure to have an orgasm*. It's important not to judge or criticize what you're doing.

And remember, there's no right or wrong way of stroking yourself. Whatever feels nice is right for you. However, you should avoid a heavy touch. Women sometimes learn to press very hard when previous attempts to have an orgasm have been "hard work." If your touch hurts, you're *definitely* pressing too hard (but if you can't feel a thing, your touch is probably too *soft*).

℘

YOU'RE NOW READY for a little fantasy. Read the description in the exercise below. Then, shut your eyes and stroke your vulva, clitoris, vagina, and other parts of your body while picturing what I describe. Enjoy the feelings that emerge as you do this.

## a little fantasy

*Imagine that your sexual feelings are like warm syrup that can flow through all parts of your body, melting away any negativity and making you feel relaxed and peaceful.*

*Shut your eyes and picture this warm syrup flowing gently through your body.*

*Feel its warmth. Feel its smoothness. Feel yourself melting and relaxing as it glides from your clitoris, through your pelvis, your legs, your arms, and to every part of your body.*

Don't forget that the aim of this exercise is to be able to focus, in a relaxed way, on the pleasure sensations created by your touch and to enjoy what you're feeling. THAT'S ALL! No other expectations are called for.

This means:

- NO analyzing of what's going on
- NO judging yourself negatively
- NO thinking about other things
- NO willing your body to orgasm

If you can do Step 3 without any discomfort, go to Step 4.

Otherwise, stay with Step 3 and do it three more times. Don't even think of going to Step 4 if you're having any difficulties completing the exercise in the way I've described.

❧

IF YOU'RE FEELING irritable or tense during the exercise, stop, and see if you can understand why. Some women react like that when they begin to enjoy their feelings of sexual pleasure. It's as if they want to stop the feelings before they get stronger. The more they enjoy the sensations, the more they tense up and try to find negative things to say about their enjoyment.

---

That sounds just like me.
I feel like I shouldn't let myself go like that,
like it's wrong or bad or something.

---

I'm sure you know, by now, that you're not alone in thinking this way. But, as you also know, that kind of thinking will turn you off in a flash unless it's quickly replaced with positive thoughts.

Look at the exercise below. I've given you several examples of positive thoughts that can be used to replace the negative ones. Say them *out loud* now to see if they feel comfortable. If they do, say them again. If not, put them into your own words and say these out loud a couple of times.

## super-positive thoughts

- I'm an adult. It's now okay for me to let my sexual feelings go.
- Being aroused and having orgasms is part of being human; it's alright for me to now enjoy my sexuality.
- I have a right to feel sexual passion.
- I can choose to let myself go whenever I feel ready.

Say the positive thoughts (yours or mine) once more, *and listen carefully to what you're saying.* When you next do the Step 3 exercise, repeat these thoughts out loud, or whisper them to yourself.

Some women get irritable during Step 3 for a different reason. They're used to touching themselves in some way other than with their fingers. Here are some examples:

- You may prefer a vibrator.
- Maybe you've always squeezed your legs together, rather than touched yourself directly on the clitoris with fingers.
- Perhaps you usually rub against something as you lie on your stomach.

None of these ways of feeling sexual is wrong. If, however, they don't allow you to feel orgasms, you probably need to find new ways of getting aroused. Although this doesn't mean you have to give away your present style of masturbating, you may have to expand it to include methods that make it easier to orgasm.

My suggestion is that you first learn how to become highly aroused using your fingers. Once you can do that, you may want to include a mixture of old and new ways of masturbating that will allow you to orgasm more easily.

**A warning:** Changing our methods of arousal can be frustrating. At first, the new method doesn't seem to give us feelings as strong as those we normally get with the old one. Don't give up. Your body has learned to get aroused with one style of masturbating, and it takes time for it to switch to another.

Tell yourself that it's useful to develop more than one way to feel sexual pleasure. After all, we're not banning vibrators or other methods— just expanding what you do to allow arousal to build to orgasm.

There are two approaches you can take with Step 3 (see also chapter 10: Habits that affect arousal). Firstly, you can continue doing the exercise as I've suggested and simply give your body time to make the adjustment. It might take a month, two months, or longer for this to happen, so don't get impatient.

Alternatively, you can combine my exercise with your masturbation style. Begin by using your way of touching yourself for one minute, then shift to using fingers for two minutes. Then, go back to the old way for another minute, before using your fingers again. Keep this up for the fifteen minutes, *but always finish with using your fingers.*

Do this on at least nine occasions. Don't forget to stroke the rest of your body and to relax and enjoy yourself.

If you'd like to change completely, just increase the time for using your fingers until gradually this method replaces your old style.

### STEP 4: allowing sexual feelings to build

Hey, we're up to Step 4! You're doing well!

In this exercise I want you to continue touching your vulva, clitoris, vagina and other parts of your body just as you did in Step 3. Move your hips and body as you touch these areas. Tighten and relax your muscles from time to time.

Focus on the sensations and feelings you get. Think of warm syrup flowing through your body. Enjoy what is happening. Relax. Do this for at least ten minutes.

**Now, we add one more thing: sexual fantasies.**

Picturing a sexual scene or story as we touch ourselves can help to build sexual feelings. That's what we're now going to do.

When you feel relaxed and ready, begin to fantasize. Shut your eyes and try to think of a sexy picture. You may imagine yourself making love to someone you know, or it may be a stranger. You may picture bodies moving in a sexy way, or run through a sexual story in your mind, imagining different scenes that lead to sexual activity. You may use the story from a romantic novel or scenes from a movie. As you fantasize, keep touching yourself in all the places that give you a pleasant feeling.

**Give yourself permission to fantasize.**

If you're worried about fantasizing, remember that fantasies are private thoughts; they don't have to be shared with anyone, unless you want to.

Before you start, take a moment to think over the fantasies you've used in the past. If you discovered that Cause #24 (Conditioning by habits and fantasies) was one of the reasons for your difficulties with orgasm, you should use the suggestions in chapter 10 for changing your fantasies.

I should mention that some women find it difficult to fantasize, whether it be a sexual fantasy or a daydream. There are many reasons for this.

You may have come from a family which encouraged children to be practical and rational, not creative and imaginative. You may have been actively discouraged from daydreaming (for example, Mom or Dad saying, *Don't sit there dreaming, there's plenty to be done*). Or, you may have spent your childhood at a computer, rather than playing make-believe and inventing your own games.

Whatever the reason, some women simply don't picture things when they're thinking.

------

That's me exactly. My mind seems to go blank if I try to imagine anything. And you can forget about fantasizing while I'm masturbating. As soon as I try to picture anything, I lose concentration and it all comes to a grinding halt.

------

Yes, I know this can happen. But you probably have talents in other directions!

⟨⟩

HOWEVER, YOU MAY be able to teach yourself to use fantasy. There are two ways to approach it.

First, rather than picture a scene, try *remembering* a romantic or sexy story you've seen, read or heard. When doing Step 4, go through the story in your mind as if you were reading a book or watching a film.

Second, you might like to try using ready-made pictures (drawings, photos, and so on) that are a sexual turn-on for you. Cut them out and look at them during the exercise, to help build your sexual arousal. If you can, memorize them and try remembering them during the exercise.

How often should you do Step 4? **For at least twenty minutes on the first four occasions, then twenty-five minutes for another four times.** This may take two or three weeks to complete.

Don't try to cram the sessions into a short period of time (unless you're really enjoying what's happening and want to do the exercise more often). It's better to space it to once every few days, so that you're looking forward to doing it. The last thing I want is for it to become a chore you feel you *have* to do.

Spacing it out also gives your mind and body time to adjust to any changes you're making.

Now, please read my next comment very carefully.

**The aim of this exercise is:**
**1. To learn how to allow your sexual feelings to become more and more intense,**
**2. while you stay relaxed and unpressured.**

You may not believe what I'm about to tell you, *but I don't want you to try to orgasm*. If it happens accidentally, don't worry. I wouldn't want you to put brakes on the feelings you get. After all, the exercise is about allowing your sexual feelings to build, not holding them back. However, it's simply not important to have an orgasm at this stage (and I certainly don't want you worrying about one).

Learning how to enjoy your sexual pleasure *as it becomes more intense* is what this exercise is all about.

Relax, then, and remember the arousal hill. You're taking a nice leisurely walk up the hill, enjoying the scenery as you go. The more relaxed you are, the easier it will be. Later, you will see the view from the top. But if you try to rush things or push yourself too hard, you'll be exhausted before you can get there.

We're so used to putting in effort to achieve things that it's easy to think sexual arousal works the same way. Well, it doesn't. In fact, the *opposite* is probably true. The more you can relax and lose yourself in the image of the warm syrup slowly gliding through your body, the more your sexual feelings will gently float to the surface of your awareness.

So, no "working hard." This isn't a test, and there's no exam to pass.

Do the exercise for *at least* the number of times I've mentioned (twenty minutes on four occasions, then twenty-five minutes on four occasions).

Experiment. Try touching yourself in different ways. Vary your fantasies. Find out what turns you on. Find out how your body changes when you're more aroused. Roll a finger backwards and forwards just above your clitoris glans and feel your clitoris shaft. Explore your G-spot, and see if it becomes sensitive. By the way, when you first stroke your G-spot, you may feel like urinating for a few seconds, but this will quickly pass.

Don't forget to gently rock your hips as you touch yourself. Loosen up and enjoy yourself.

Try making sounds that express your pleasure. Learning to let go in this way can help you to relax and allow the feelings to build.

Notice how your sexual feelings come and go. Even as they become stronger, you'll notice they sometimes level off, or slide into a valley. This is quite natural. Just keep touching and fantasizing, and the feelings will slowly begin to build again.

**Be prepared to stay in this situation while your feelings grow stronger.**

You'll have to be the judge of whether you're ready to move on to the next step. If you feel your arousal levels becoming stronger and stronger (more intense than you're used to), *and* you're nicely relaxed and not pushing yourself about having to orgasm, then go to Step 5. If not, keep doing the exercise until you've met these conditions.

It doesn't matter whether you do Step 4 on ten or fifty occasions. As I said, this isn't a test. You won't get a gold medal for taking the least number of times to do the exercise, but you could give yourself a pat on the back if you continue to practice for the length of time that you need.

℘

WHAT DO YOU do if your sexual feelings start to lessen? Take a moment to think about how *you* could have made this happen. Did you have a negative thought? Did you become tense? Did some emotion fill your stomach or chest? Did you start to think about some task you need to do later? Were you distracted by something or someone?

Take some time to identify how you may have switched yourself off sexually. If the distraction was not of your doing, see if you can change things so that it doesn't happen again. If it's your own thinking that led to sexual shut-down, go back to the Super-Positive Thoughts. I've repeated them below. Try to return to the positive thinking you had before.

## super-positive thoughts

- I'm an adult. It's now okay for me to let my sexual feelings go.
- Being aroused and having orgasms is part of being human; it's alright for me to now enjoy my sexuality.
- I have a right to feel sexual passion.
- I can choose to let myself go whenever I feel ready.

When you feel ready, return to the exercise and start again. Begin by lying there quietly and saying the Super-Positive Thoughts to yourself or out loud. Say them several times, listening carefully to what you're saying.

At this point, check out how you feel. Do you feel stronger, more in control? Then begin the exercise again, keeping the Super-Positive Thoughts at the back of your mind. Whenever you feel the need, stop and repeat them until you feel more positive.

However, if you're still having difficulties, open your eyes, sit up, and take some time to think about what's happening.

Do you need to work harder at ridding yourself of negative thoughts? Do you need to take further action to stop the interruptions? Is there something you can do to make yourself more relaxed? What do you need to get yourself in the right mood? How can you stop pressuring yourself with expectations? How can you become less upset/anxious/afraid?

Make whatever changes you can to help yourself enjoy the exercise. Don't feel you have to do this on your own. You may be able to enlist the help of your partner. See a psychologist or sexual therapist if you're feeling stuck. And, most importantly,

**BE PATIENT.**

The point of breaking this Program into small steps is that it provides you with the chance of finding out exactly where the problem lies. Each step can bring up issues that make you uncomfortable. Recognize that you've done well to come this far. The problems you're now having in Step 4 offer you the chance to stop and ask, *What is it about THIS part of the Program that is difficult for me?* Finding the answer to that question can help you to move on.

When you feel ready to return to the exercise, try again.

At this point you may find it helpful to use a vibrator to assist in building your arousal. The movement of a vibrator is strong and regular. This can often help to override turn-off messages.

However, try not to use a vibrator all the way through the exercise. If used too long, it can easily make your clitoris feel numb. Begin with your fingers. If you get to a point where your sexual feelings seem to go no further, switch to the vibrator. As you feel your arousal begin to build again, try switching back to using your fingers. Switch backwards and forwards in this way until you finish the exercise. But, *always* end the exercise by using your fingers.

### STEP 5: letting go of control

In Step 4 you learned how to relax and let your sexual arousal build to higher levels than you've felt before. Slowly you've been letting go of the need to control your sexual feelings.

It's now time to let yourself climb to the top of the arousal hill and enjoy the view. You're almost there. All it needs is for you to let go just that little bit more.

In Step 5 continue to do everything you were doing in Step 4.

Stay relaxed, focus only on the sexual feelings and, except for sexual fantasies, keep your thoughts focused on *you*. Enjoy the feelings of pleasure and allow them to gradually fill every part of your body. From time to time, tighten and relax your pelvic muscles in a steady rhythm. Use your vibrator if you need to, but in the way I described earlier.

**Don't try to force your feelings. Let them lead you.**

Have confidence that your arousal will take you through to orgasm—if you let it.

Before you begin touching yourself sexually, let's see how prepared you are to let go of control. The following exercise should help you. So, find somewhere private and quiet to lie or sit and imagine the following picture. *Don't read further until you've done the exercise on the next page.*

# imagine

*Imagine it's a delightful sunny day. You're walking along a path you've never been on before, a path edged with beautiful flowers and shrubs. Colorful birds flit through the trees. You go deeper and deeper into the forest, until you realize you're unsure of where you are.*

*Imagine that in front of you appears a bright shaft of light, showing you the way back. If you follow the light, you cannot get lost. There's no need to think about what's happening. All you have to do is follow.*

*So, follow the light and notice what happens.*

How did you go? Did you allow yourself to follow the instructions and go with the light? Or did you struggle, wanting to know where you're going, or needing to be in control?

If you can allow yourself to go with the light, then begin doing Step 5. Take the same attitude you had about following the light, and turn it towards your sexual arousal. Follow your feelings and trust them to take you in the right direction. Let them take you to feelings of greater and greater pleasure. Trust your body to know its own direction, and it will take you to the top of your arousal hill. All you have to do is enjoy the scenery as you go. You don't have to lead. You don't have to know where you're going. For once, you can let go.

Each time you do Step 5, begin with the image of the path and with you allowing yourself to be led by the light. Then begin touching your body, and follow the sexual feelings up the pathway that leads to the top of the mountain (now what a great fantasy that could become!).

Remember to stay relaxed. Trust your body to lead you. And don't forget the most important thing: to enjoy your pleasure as it builds stronger and stronger.

**Continue to do the exercise each week** (*at least* once a week) and, one day, you'll find your feelings becoming strong enough to carry you along the path to orgasm.

How will this feel?

It may seem like tiny fireworks are exploding briefly inside you. Or it may feel as if a whole fireworks display is lighting up your body.

As you become more practiced at letting yourself go, the feelings will grow more intense and may last longer.

Don't be surprised if your body moves or twitches a little; this is just your muscles tightening. Remember, during orgasm it's the pulsing of the muscles that is partly responsible for the pleasurable feelings. You may also find yourself breathing faster for a few moments and your skin becoming a little clammy as you perspire. All of these reactions are perfectly natural.

**You were born with the ability to feel orgasms, and your body is responding just as it should.**

Within a few moments, though, you'll find everything will quiet down again—except now you should be feeling quite peaceful and relaxed. PLEASE, just lie there and enjoy this special feeling for a few moments.

If you find that orgasm happens when you use the vibrator, that's great. After you can do this several times, try using the vibrator to build your arousal until you're very close to orgasm, then switch to your fingers. This will help you to feel confident that *you* can give yourself an orgasm, rather than thinking it's all the work of the vibrator.

℗

NOW, LET ME return to those of you who had difficulty imagining yourself being led by the light. Take some time to think about why this is so. Are you a person who likes to be in control at all times? Are you someone who gets nervous about the unknown? Are you a very practical person, who feels silly imagining something that isn't *real*? In other words, is your difficulty telling you something about the way you approach life?

During earlier chapters in this book, you probably began to think about how your personality and style affected your sexual arousal patterns. So you may not be surprised by your reaction to the *path-and-light* fantasy. At this point, take some time to explore this further. If necessary, seek help from an experienced therapist. See if you can learn to let go of the need to be in control.

Then try the path-and-light fantasy again on two more occasions. If you can follow it more easily, continue with the masturbation exercise as I've described above. If you simply can't go with the path-and-light fantasy, then replace it with some positive statements such as:

- All I need to do is relax and follow where my feelings take me.
- I don't have to lead the way, only enjoy the feelings.

Say these statements to yourself for a few moments, before beginning to touch your body. If you start to tense up or try to take control, pause and repeat the statements, listening carefully to the meaning of the words. Continue doing the exercise in this way.

How often do you do Step 5? For as long as you need. Some women may begin to feel orgasms after ten or so sessions, carried out over several weeks. Others will find they need a few months. Every woman is different. So, there's no point wishing your body and mind would react more quickly than they do. You are who you are. Don't put pressure on yourself at this stage.

You may find, after having an orgasm the first time, that you can't seem to get so aroused the next time you try.

But I thought that once I started having orgasms, I wouldn't have to worry any more.

Sometimes it's like that. However, for many women, having their first orgasm (or learning to orgasm again) is so exciting that they rush back the next day to try again—and try *too hard*. And, you know what that will do, don't you? Sexual feelings just can't be forced.

Be prepared, then, to continue with Step 5, knowing you *can* orgasm and in time will do so again. It might help to think that what you're doing is learning a new skill. After all, discovering how to relax, enjoy sexual pleasure, and allow your arousal to build to levels needed for orgasm *is* a skill. And just as learning how to use a computer, ride a bike or paint in oils needs a lot of practice before these skills come naturally, so, too, does learning to have orgasms.

# combining the personal and couple change programs |

ONCE YOU'VE BEGUN to orgasm, you may feel ready to start the Couple Change Program. However, don't stop your own Program as outlined in this chapter. It's important to keep practicing. This will increase your understanding of how to arouse yourself. It will also help to develop your confidence in being able to orgasm.

Of course, there's no pressure to get together with your partner just yet. Continue with the Personal Change Program for as long as you feel the need. Keep talking to your partner about what's happening, and be clear that you're not yet ready to start the Couple Program.

For those who don't have a partner at the moment and want to develop more confidence in having orgasms when they *do*, it's possible to go through the Couple Change Program in your imagination. Read through each step and then imagine doing it with a partner. You might be surprised at how helpful this can be (not to mention fun).

# 14

# learning to orgasm
## with a partner
### the couple change program

IN AN EARLIER chapter, I mentioned that many women have been taught to please others before themselves. They worry about how they look, whether they're too sexy (or not sexy enough), whether their partner is having his or her sexual needs met, and so on. In fact, they often give so much attention to pleasing a partner during sex that their own feelings of pleasure are ignored.

---

But isn't that the whole point of having sex with a partner—to give sexual pleasure to another person?

---

Well, I agree that helping our partner to feel sexual pleasure is one of the reasons for having sex with a partner. But, the *whole point*? I don't think so. Actually, women have sex with another person for many different reasons. Here are some examples:

## some reasons for having sex with a partner

- to feel close
- to feel loved
- to show a partner you love him/her
- to end an argument
- to express a sexual urge
- for relaxation
- to give pleasure to a partner
- to enjoy your sexual arousal
- for money
- to prove you're attractive
- to relieve stress
- to prove you're worthwhile
- to prove you can be seductive
- to keep the peace
- to be physically touched
- because you're forced into it
- to feel less lonely
- to fulfill a duty
- other (write down any others that fit you)

---

In other words, sex can include meeting your needs as well as your partner's. Actually, sex *must* be about pleasing yourself if you want to orgasm.

**To help your arousal build to orgasm, you must be able to concentrate on your sexual pleasure.**

Of course, I'm not suggesting you go to the other extreme and focus only on *your* arousal and forget about your partner's needs.

Putting *all* your attention on yourself or on your partner isn't the answer. *There has to be a balance between the two.* This is easier said than done. Being aware of how you're feeling and, at the same time, noticing what's happening with your partner can be tricky.

# the advantages of
# the couple change program |

THE COUPLE CHANGE Program is designed to help you find this balance so that you can orgasm more easily. It also:

- teaches you how to move from having an orgasm on *your* own to having one with your partner
- is a relaxing way to become close to your partner again
- gives you a chance to talk more openly about sex with your partner
- teaches you to feel comfortable giving attention to your sexual arousal and needs
- teaches you to move attention from your sexual feelings to those of your partner—and back again
- teaches you to make time for the sexual side of your relationship

In fact, many couples I've worked with continue doing the Program long after they've finished the last exercise. They say it's fun, pleasurable and relaxing—and a great way to get into lovemaking.

# concerns about doing
# the couple change program |

I'M SURE SOME of you are feeling a little nervous about doing a sexual program with your partner. Don't worry if you are. Many women feel this way. Let's look at why you might be worried.

- **Worries about yourself:**
  - You feel uncomfortable talking openly about your orgasm difficulties with your partner.
  - Since doing the Personal Change Program, you now

orgasm more easily, but lack confidence that you can do so with your partner.

- You're not yet confident of your ability to have an orgasm and wonder whether it's too early to try with your partner.
- You're not happy with the shape of your body or your genitals and feel that the Program will expose the way you look.
- You're afraid that if the Program doesn't help, you'll be a failure.

- **Worries about your partner:**
  - You're worried your partner won't treat the Program seriously.
  - You're afraid your partner will get bored.
  - You're scared your partner will use the Program as a chance to have sex.
  - You're afraid your partner will get angry about having to take time from other activities.

- **Worries about practical matters:**
  - You're not sure how you'll get the time to do the Program.
  - You're afraid you'll never get the privacy to do it.
  - You believe the physical disabilities/conditions that you or your partner have could make it hard to get through the Program.

Now, take some time to think through your concerns. Is there any evidence to back them up, or are they really fears of what *might* happen?

If there *is* good reason for your worries, try talking with your partner to see if you can change something in the situation, so that you'll feel happier. While many practical problems can be sorted out, occasionally some can't. For example, if you and your partner are still living with parents, privacy on a regular basis may be impossible. In that case, you may have to do the Program at a later date.

If you've been making yourself anxious with what might happen (you know, *what if he/she doesn't like. . . ? what if I can't. . . ?*—and so on), then you should also talk with your partner. He or she may have no idea of what's troubling you. A chat could ease your mind.

Talk. Don't bottle up your feelings. Otherwise, your imagination will start to run wild, and everything will seem a hundred times worse. Hopefully, talking with your partner will help to reduce your fears.

Of course, this is easier when you have a good relationship. If your relationship isn't going as well as you'd like, it might be tempting to avoid having that chat, for fear of rocking the boat.

---

But, we've just started getting on again. Why risk losing the peacefulness we have at the moment? Couldn't I sort out my fears on my own?

---

Yes, you could try to do that. You might even talk them through with a therapist. But, just remember, if you don't tackle your concerns, they'll eventually bubble their way to the surface—probably while you're doing the Program. This will certainly let your partner know there's something worrying you. However, the force of your outburst may also set back any progress you've made. Better to bring everything out in the open now, when you have time to get your thoughts in order first.

By the way, many women find they become less worried once they start the Couple Change Program. It's not as difficult as they imagined and a lot more enjoyable than they expected.

## start the couple change program when . . .

NOW LET ME talk to those of you whose relationship is not going well. You may have found that your partner doesn't want to listen to concerns about your orgasm difficulties. Or that he or she doesn't want to read through this chapter with you. What do you do? It's very simple.

**Don't do the Program . . . yet!**

Save yourself the heartache. You can't do it on your own. And without a partner's support, you'll only become *more* worried about the outcome. WITH GOOD REASON. So get some help. See a good relationship therapist—with your partner, if possible. It's better to come back to the Couple Change Program later, when you both have a more positive attitude. In the meantime, keep on with your own Personal Change Program.

In fact, it's not just the willingness of your partner that you need to check out. There are several conditions to be met before you begin the Program. Read the list below and place a check next to those that apply at this time:

❐ Both you and your partner really want to do it.
❐ Your partner is interested enough to read about the Program.
❐ You are both prepared to follow the Program as outlined.
❐ You are both committed to making the time to do the exercises.
❐ You are both able to express physical affection (nonsexual) towards each other.
❐ You both feel physically attracted to each other.
❐ You both want the relationship to continue.
❐ You both feel emotional fondness for each other (you don't have to be madly in love).
❐ You feel ready to have an orgasm with your partner (even if you're not entirely comfortable with the idea).

Based on the number of checks, decide whether you're ready to do the Program. Be honest with yourself. Talk it over with your partner. See if he or she agrees with you. If you feel too many conditions are missing, delay doing it.

The more you can meet these conditions, the greater the likelihood of the Program being helpful and enjoyable. If necessary, wait until you're ready to make it work. See a psychologist or relationship therapist, if you need help.

Did you notice I haven't suggested that you need to be *confident* about your abilities or even *convinced* that the Program will work?

These are not necessary to begin. However, there is one final condition that MUST be met:

❑ **You are prepared to *try* the Program and to put in as much effort as you can.**

Can you meet this last condition? I hope so.

# getting ready to begin |

BEFORE YOU START, there are a few things to think about.

## 1. Plan when you'll be doing the exercises.

You'll need to do three exercises a week, or five over two weeks. And each one lasts an hour. This means a bit of planning is needed before you start. Work out your available times and jot a note into your diary or calendar. That way, you'll stop yourself from filling each week with other things. If work and family commitments or medical conditions make it impossible to do the exercises this often, do still plan ahead as much as possible. If something comes up unexpectedly and you have to change the exercise time, decide on the new time slot as quickly as possible.

By the way, there will probably be occasions when you feel annoyed or upset with your partner and not in the mood for the Program. If this happens, it's better to do the exercise on another day when you're both feeling happier with each other.

Remember, the longer you take to do the exercises, the slower may be the progress. There's nothing wrong with that. But you'll need to be realistic and not expect too much too soon.

## 2. Make the Program a priority.

Tell yourself it's important and can't be put off. *I know, I know,* you already have every waking moment filled with something to do. Well then, be prepared to cancel things or change arrangements. You may have to stop some other tasks or activities for a while, to give you more time. Keep in mind that this is time for you and your relationship. The Program is an *investment in your future happiness*. Make it count.

### 3. Find some private space to do the exercises.

You won't relax if there are other people wandering around outside the room in which you're doing the Program. Try to make your time together as private as possible. Women can be easily distracted from their sexual feelings, so there's no point starting an exercise if all your attention is on what's happening on the other side of the door.

Unfortunately, waiting until midnight when everyone is asleep probably isn't such a good idea. Sleeping during the exercise doesn't make any sense, either!

Make sure the room is heated or cooled to make it comfortable to do the exercise. If your partner's body temperature is different from yours, take some time to work out what you can do about this (for example, place the heater closer to the person who feels the cold).

### 4. Take a shower or bath before you begin.

You won't be able to relax during the massage if you're worried about body odor.

The Program is done with your clothes off, but if you feel uncomfortable with that, wear panties for the first step, until you relax.

Bathing offers a good chance to slow down your thinking and relax. It also gives you time to switch from being busy wife, mother, employee, gardener (or any other role you've been in that day) to lover and partner. You certainly won't enjoy the exercises if you're unable to make the switch. Spending some relaxing time with your partner before beginning the massage can also help you to switch to lover/partner.

## 5. Treat the Program as a new start.

Try to let the past go, and see the Program as a way of starting over again. Think positive and don't assume that past problems caused by your orgasm difficulties will occur again (remember how damaging negative attitudes can be). Try to look forward, not backwards.

## 6. See the Program as your special time together.

Set the tone by lighting a few candles, dimming the lights and choosing some quiet music to play in the background. Whatever you do, avoid treating the Program as a chore. Otherwise, you might as well go back to watching TV.

## 7. Don't pressure yourself with expectations.

I know this may be difficult for women who like to set goals, but the Program is designed to *reduce* the pressure to have an orgasm (while at the same time helping you to orgasm more easily!). Do your bit, then, and try to keep your expectations in check. Just relax and follow the Program as described. Don't try to figure out (control) what's going to happen; simply allow your feelings to flow at their own pace.

## 8. Don't give up at the first obstacle.

It's quite normal to feel a little anxious at the beginning of each new step in the Program. This should change, however, as you do the exercise a second, third or more times. Soon you'll begin to relax and enjoy what's happening. By the way, check how your partner is feeling. He or she may also be a little anxious.

If other negative emotions or thoughts pop up, *always* take the time to sort them out with your partner (or a therapist) before starting the next step of the Program. Never try to force yourself to go on. Your emotions and thoughts are telling you there's a problem somewhere that is affecting your sexual well-being.

Events or medical problems might also stop you from completing some step of the Program. Don't pressure yourself to finish the exercise (or Program) simply because you've started it. Wait until you've sorted out the difficulty or obstacle, and then begin again.

**9. Make allowances for physical conditions that restrict you.**

If you have a disability or physical condition, be prepared to adapt the exercises to your needs. There's no point being uncomfortable or in pain. Use your imagination to change the position or activity, and ask your partner to help. At the same time, try to understand the point of each step and keep to it as much as possible. And remember, there's no gold medal for pushing ahead regardless.

# what is the couple change program?

THE PROGRAM IS made up of a set of exercises to be done each week. It begins with some gentle massaging that slowly becomes more and more sexual with each new step.

You'll give a massage and also receive one during the one-hour exercise. Don't panic if you've never done this before. You don't need any massaging experience to do the Program.

Actually, what you'll be doing is really an exercise in *pleasuring*. By gently massaging or stroking your partner, you can *give* a feeling of sensual pleasure. At the same time, you'll have the chance to feel or receive pleasure through the touch of fingers on skin. When the roles are reversed, you'll be the one to feel the pleasure of being stroked, and your partner can enjoy the sensation of doing this to you.

There is, however, one important condition for doing the Program that I haven't mentioned before:

**While you do it, the exercises will replace your usual sexual activities.**

Other than the touching and activity allowed during the Program, any other sexual touching between you and your partner (both during the massage and at other times) needs to stop. Of course, you can always hug and be physically affectionate in a *nonsexual* way.

Oops, I can almost hear some of you gasping!

---

Well, it's a bit of a shock to hear you say that. I'm
fine with it, but I'm not sure how my husband would
feel about it.

---

I understand your concern. Let me explain. You won't actually be without any sexual activity during the Program. In fact, with each step the massaging becomes more and more sexual in touch.

It's very important, however, that you stick to what is described for each exercise. There's a good reason for this. For many women with orgasm difficulties, sex has become a stressful activity. They often try to avoid sex with their partner because of this, and may even stop hugging and kissing.

What you need is the chance to feel *positive* towards lovemaking, not negative. The sensual massaging offers this chance. It puts you into a setting similar to the sexual setting you're used to, but without the pressure of having to feel sexual arousal or orgasm.

When you begin the Couple Change Program, *there are no expectations for you to feel sexual*. If you do feel aroused, that's fine. If you don't, that's also fine. Without any sexual demands to be met, you'll be amazed at how easy it is to relax and enjoy your partner's company.

---

You're right. I can remember how nice lovemaking
was before I got hung up on trying to have an
orgasm. Not having to worry about what's going to
happen—it feels like a weight's been lifted off my
shoulders!

---

Many women feel the same way. Some don't even realize how burdened they've been feeling until they begin the first step of the Program. Suddenly, there's nothing they have to *do* sexually, and it feels wonderful.

But, please, don't try to stop any feelings of sexual pleasure that might arise during the massage. I certainly don't want you to develop any *new* guilt complexes. Remember, there's nothing wrong with feeling aroused. It's straining to get aroused and to orgasm that's the problem.

Let me now describe each stage of the Program in detail. Hopefully, you're keen to get started.

# the couple change program |

BEFORE YOU BEGIN, let me make a STRONG suggestion that you read one step of the Program, and *then do it, before reading about the next step.* When you feel ready to move on, then read about the next step. Otherwise, you may get nervous wondering whether you'll be able to complete the later steps.

Each step follows on from the other. When you can do one step, the next one should follow naturally. But, if you were to jump straight into Step 5, for example, it would probably seem difficult. So, do it the easy way: take one step at a time.

## STEP 1: sensual massage

### Let's set the scene

You'll need to find a place where you can be private for at least an hour. Turn the answering machine on and don't answer the door. The last thing you need is a stream of interruptions.

Make sure the area where you'll be doing the massage is comfortable. You'll be lying flat for thirty minutes when you're being massaged. And when giving the massage you'll be kneeling or sitting beside your partner. Some people do the Program on their bed while others lie on a mattress on the floor (perhaps in front of the fire).

Place a towel on the bed. You may want to use massage oil or talcum powder to make it easier for your hands to slide over your partner's skin, so you'll need to protect the mattress. Have a spare towel nearby. During the massage, you're lying still and your body may cool down. If necessary, use the spare towel to cover those parts of your body not being massaged.

Check the temperature of the room. If it's too cool, bring in some heating. If it's too hot, find some way to cool things down.

If you enjoy music, you may like to have some playing quietly in the background. However, choose some without words; otherwise, you'll find yourself singing the chorus, and not paying attention to the massage.

Make the atmosphere romantic by lighting candles or dimming the lights. Just make sure you can easily see each other. This isn't an exercise in hide-and-seek.

**What do we do?**

In this exercise you'll be massaging each other in turn, with your hands and fingers. Each time you do the exercise, one of you will be massaged first and when this is finished, you'll switch and the other person will be massaged. However, for this first step, some parts of the body are "banned." I'm sure you can guess which parts I mean. They are:

- Breasts and nipples (men as well as women—we have to keep it fair!)
- Buttocks (bottom, butt)
- Genitals

This applies to both you and your partner. Since I've sometimes heard men groan at this, I should point out that this still leaves *most* of the body to be massaged.

You have thirty minutes each which, of course, means fifteen minutes for each side of the body. I don't want you to feel you must watch the clock and finish exactly on time. Still, the timing is important. Five minutes each side is too rushed and an hour would be too tiring. After the first few massages, you'll be able to judge the time and won't need to keep an eye on the clock.

Choose who's going to be massaged first. Just one thing: make sure that whoever is really tired does *not* go first. Otherwise, he or she might find it impossible to get up in order to massage the other person. By the way, for the same reason avoid doing the massage late at night (unless you're both night owls).

Try to vary the time of doing the exercise. You might try an afternoon on one occasion, a morning during a day off work, or nights during the week.

Always start the massage by lying on your stomach. Women often feel vulnerable when they're lying on their back, so it's easier to start this way. When your back (minus buttocks) has been massaged, turn over so your front can be massaged (excluding breasts, nipples, and genitals).

After the first person has been massaged, give him or her a few moments to slowly sit up, and then switch over. You could use this time to change the music or go to the toilet.

∾

NOW, LET ME say something about the style of massage used. As I've already mentioned, you don't have to know anything about massage to be able to do this exercise.

Just use a gentle stroking or caressing action with your hands. Touch the way *you'd* like to be touched during lovemaking. *Don't* try to imitate a sports masseur. *Don't* try to do a deep body massage. This is supposed to be a sensuous enjoyable experience, not a painful one! Use the massage oil (or talcum powder) to make your hands run easily over your partner's skin.

As you're being massaged, close your eyes and put your attention onto the place you're being touched. Don't *think about* the massage. Just notice the feelings you get from your partner's stroking. And, check out which parts of your body are more (or less) sensitive than other parts. In other words, use this time to learn about yourself.

If you have a physical condition or disability that prevents much, or any, feeling in some parts of your body, you may find that *other* parts have become more sensitive. Check this out.

**You'll need to do three massages over a week, or five over two weeks.**

During the first two of these, the person *being* massaged should tell their partner when they're enjoying the touch. They should also say when the massage feels uncomfortable—and why. If necessary, *show* your partner what kind of touch you like. Everyone likes a slightly different touch, so be prepared to learn what your partner likes and doesn't like, and use that knowledge in future massages. After all, there's no point touching your partner in a way that he or she finds irritating.

By the way, if you get ticklish, ask your partner to massage a little more heavily where you feel it most. Keep in mind, too, that being a little nervous can also make you ticklish. As you get used to the exercise and relax, you'll probably find the ticklishness disappears.

If you have a physical condition or disability, you may need to think about adapting where and how you do the massage. Use cushions, heated mattresses, water beds, or whatever will make you more comfortable. Raise your shoulders or lie on your side if need be. You may need to allow a little longer for the exercise. Or you may find it too tiring to do it for the time I've suggested.

If you sometimes get muscle spasms, try not to become anxious about it. This isn't the movies, where no one finds crumbs in the bed or gets a cramp in their leg or knocks over the massage oil. Real life is about things not always working out the way we'd want them to. So, if a spasm breaks the mood of the massage, take a short break, and continue when you're ready.

### The point of it all

---

This all sounds great. But what am I supposed to be doing while the massage is going on? Make polite conversation with my partner?

---

Just close your eyes and direct all your attention to the area being touched. Try to *feel* where you're being touched. Don't think *about* what's happening, just be aware. Don't analyze, simply feel the touch and enjoy it. And, no chatting—it will only distract you.

During this exercise (and the whole Program), try to put your attention on what is happening at the moment. To use a popular expression, *stay in the present.* That means:

- NO shopping lists going through your mind
- NO discussions about the kids during the massage
- NO worrying about orgasms
- NO judging

- And of course, NO singing along to the music (wait until later, when you're in the shower).

This is a pleasuring exercise, remember. Give your mind a rest and allow yourself to feel the pleasure of being gently stroked.

If that's difficult, try saying the word "relax," while you're being massaged. Remember to breathe evenly and deeply.

### Getting turned on

---

I know it doesn't matter if I get turned on or not, but I'm worried about what will happen if I do get sexually aroused? You said there's to be no sexual touching with my partner.

---

That's right. So, for the first few steps (later there will be touching), you have three options. The first option is to have a cold shower (just kidding). The second option is to allow your feelings to just fade away. Interestingly, women find this easier to do than men, who have learned that, once aroused, they should have an orgasm.

The third option is the most interesting because it's one that women don't often think about. After both massages are finished, you can touch *yourself* while your partner (perhaps doing the same thing) lies beside you. I know some women have not done this before. Let me tell you why I think it's a good idea.

It can be very important for couples to feel comfortable enough with each other to be able to masturbate (themselves, not each other) while lying side by side. If you're in a long-term relationship, there's going to be some occasion in the future when one of you feels sexually aroused and the other doesn't. One of you may be very stressed at work. One of you may have a medical condition. One of you may be putting all your energies into a project or passing exams. And so on. Situations like these can easily stop us from feeling sexual.

Rather than feeling resentful or having to bottle up sexual feelings, I believe it's better to become comfortable masturbating with your partner cuddling up beside you. It's amazing how much closer you'll both feel.

This is why I'm suggesting you be prepared to touch yourself at the end of the massage. The Program gives you the perfect opportunity to learn to do this comfortably, so you might want to consider taking it.

Don't worry if at first you feel a little embarrassed about trying this. Many women feel the same way. But after doing it once or twice, they find it rather exciting and even liberating.

If, then, you feel aroused at the end of this exercise, try telling your partner. Say you'd like to touch yourself. He or she may be feeling the same way. Lie *beside* each other. You can hold hands or touch in a nonsexual way. But *you*, not your partner, should touch your genitals, breasts, and any other areas you see as "sexual."

If you are happy to try this, let me say something about *expectations.* If you've already learned to orgasm with the Personal Change Program, do not pressure yourself to try to have an orgasm now as you lie beside your partner. You may still have difficulty letting your arousal build when you're not on your own. There'll be plenty of time for that later in this Program. Simply enjoy your feelings of sexual pleasure.

My advice is the same if you've never had problems becoming highly aroused on your own, but can't orgasm with a partner. Let the Couple Change Program teach you. For now, relax and use masturbation after the exercises to simply enjoy your sexual pleasure, rather than trying to orgasm. First, learn to become less self-conscious about being turned on in front of your partner.

If you're too uncomfortable to touch yourself after finishing Step 1, that's fine. It's not necessary to the Program, so don't worry. Perhaps you'll feel like trying in later Steps.

One more point on touching yourself. If you've been used to a vibrator and want to learn how to enjoy sexual arousal by touching with your fingers, you may need to adopt a strategy of gradually shifting from one to the other. To learn how to do this, read my earlier suggestions in chapter 10 and chapter 13 (Step 3). Of course, if you wish to continue using a vibrator, this, too, is acceptable.

**Moving on**

If you can do Step 1 without problems, go to the next exercise. If you feel the need to repeat the first exercise once or twice more, then do so. It's important to feel relaxed about what you're doing before moving on.

If doing Step 1 has made you quite uncomfortable, then take some time to think about why this might be so. Check out your thoughts. Do you have any negative ideas going through your head? Are you worrying about whether the Program will work? Are you concerned your partner is getting impatient and won't want to go on to Step 2? Do you feel uncomfortable about getting aroused? Do you feel uncomfortable by the physical closeness? What emotions do you feel? Fear? Boredom? Impatience?

Is there any need to think and feel the way you do? Perhaps old negative thoughts and emotions are coming to the surface and you need to deal with them. Reading the Super-Positive Thoughts in the box below could help you to do this. Say them *out loud*—several times.

## super-positive thoughts

- I'm an adult. It's now okay for me to let my sexual feelings go.
- Being aroused and having orgasms is part of being human. It's alright for me to now enjoy my sexuality.
- I have a right to feel sexual passion.
- I can choose to let myself go whenever I feel ready.

Perhaps your concerns relate to your partner. Sometimes women complain that their partner didn't follow the conditions of the exercise (for example, stroked too close to their genitals or breasts) and made them anxious.

If this happened, tell your partner about it. You may find that he or she thought they were doing exactly as asked. Or it may be that the exercise conditions *were* being ignored. If so, explain that you need to be able to *trust* that the exercise will be followed correctly. In fact, there are several emotions you will need to feel if you're to enjoy the exercise:

- trust
- respect
- caring
- understanding

Without these you'll find it hard to relax. The Program will then be impossible to do. Of course, your partner needs to experience them, too.

If your difficulties continue, get some help from a psychologist or relationship therapist. Don't be too discouraged. Starting the Couple Change Program can sometimes raise personal or relationship issues that didn't seem a problem before you began. If your difficulties with Step 1 seem bigger than they should be, there's probably some important issue you need to sort out first. Get some help.

## STEP 2: sensual massage—add breasts, nipples, and buttocks

This exercise is exactly the same as Step 1, except that now you can include breasts, nipples (men and women) and buttocks (but *not* genitals) when massaging.

Once again, do the exercise **three times over a week or five times over two weeks.** Don't forget to put on some music and dim the lights to set a romantic or pleasant mood.

Relax and focus on the feelings you get as you touch and are touched. Let yourself feel pampered. Forget the rest of the world. For now, there's just you and the enjoyment of the touch.

**Remember, the aim of the exercise is to allow yourself to relax and focus on the sensations of being touched.**

You should have no other expectations.

Breathe deeply and evenly as you give your attention to where you're being touched. Be aware of those parts of your body that are more sensitive than others.

If your partner isn't touching you in a pleasurable way, remember to speak up. Take this chance to explain how you like to be touched on your breasts and buttocks. Some women, for example, find their breasts are very sensitive and need a gentle touch. Make sure your partner knows this.

If you or your partner feels sexually aroused at the end of the massage, you may want to masturbate as in Step 1. Remember, the aim of this is to enjoy feelings of sexual pleasure, not to orgasm.

If you finish Step 2 without problems, then move to Step 3. If, on the other hand, the exercises have upset you in any way, do not move on yet. Take the time to understand why you're feeling this way. Women usually become upset at this stage for the reasons I've outlined below:

- They can't allow themselves to relax enough to enjoy the massage.
- They feel guilty about enjoying the massage.
- They can't stop thinking about tasks that need doing.
- They think this is progressing too slowly.
- Having their breasts touched reminds them of past sexual abuse.
- They feel self-conscious about the shape or size of their breasts or buttocks.
- They think they should be feeling sexual arousal now that their breasts and buttocks are being touched.
- They're annoyed that a disability stops them from doing the massage for the full hour.
- They feel uncomfortable with not knowing what is supposed to happen.
- They're worried their partner seems to be losing interest in doing the Program.
- Their partner touched them on the genitals and laughed when they got upset.
- Their partner doesn't touch them the way they've asked.

It's not uncommon for Step 2 to raise these kinds of issues. Do any of them fit you? Take some time to think it through. Talk to your partner. Get help from a therapist. Most importantly, don't give up. You may be surprised at how easily some of these problems can be sorted out.

Repeat Step 2 until you're completely comfortable with it. Trying to push on to the next step before you're ready is not a good idea. You'll put more pressure on yourself—and the result will be even *more* discomfort.

## STEP 3: massaging the complete body

In this step, while continuing to do the massage exercise just as you did before, you include the outer genital area (vulva, clitoris, entrance of the vagina, perineum, and anus).

Please note, I said, "included." You don't start or end with the genitals, but gently stroke them as you reach that area. The touch used should be the same as for other parts of the body. And the time spent on the genital area should be no longer than for other areas.

Make sure you let your partner know when you enjoy (or don't enjoy) the touch you're getting to your genitals. You did this earlier when other parts of your body were being massaged. It should be no different when it's your genitals.

If you feel a little uncomfortable with including the anus, you may leave this area out. Perhaps you'll feel more relaxed and be able to include this in the next step.

If you have a physical condition or disability which leaves you unable to feel anything when your vulva or clitoris are touched, you can choose whether to include these areas as part of the massage or not. But don't forget that surrounding areas (for example, your anus) may still be sensitive.

You are now aiming to give and receive sensual pleasure to the whole body. But please note

**... you are not trying to deliberately arouse your partner sexually or to force yourself to be aroused.**

This *may* happen because of the pleasantness of the touch. But there is no expectation of how much sexual arousal should be felt. Just stay relaxed and enjoy whatever feelings you have. On some days, these feelings may be pleasant but non-sexual. On other days, you may experience enjoyable sexual pleasure.

This is also a great time to learn more about your partner's genital area. Couples don't often take the time to stop and look. They know what their partner's face, hands, and shoulders look like—but not their genitals. So, when you're massaging, take the time to explore and learn.

Try different kinds of touch, and find out which seem to give the most pleasure. Don't be afraid to check with your partner. He or she will be pleased that you're interested enough to ask.

When it's your turn to be massaged, be aware of how you feel as your genitals are being stroked.

---

And what am I supposed to do
while he's staring at me?
I know I'd feel embarrassed.

---

Yes, you probably would. But I was just going to say that learning about our partner's genitals doesn't mean we *stare* or *peer* at them. At least, not if we want to stay popular! Just be natural, acting as you would when massaging any other part of the body.

As your body is being massaged, imagine that your feelings of pleasure (both sexual and sensual) are warm syrup flowing through every part of your body. Enjoy the warmth as it flows gently through your pelvis and stomach, up to your chest, into your arms and head, down your back, and down your legs.

Imagine that as it flows through each part of your body, any negative thoughts and feelings are gently pushed aside. Feel this warm syrup filling every part of you. Stay relaxed as you feel yourself opening up to the pleasant sensations you're experiencing. Enjoy—that's all you have to do.

Try moving gently as you're being massaged. Rock your hips with the movement of your partner's hands. Try making sounds to match how you feel.

After you've finished each massage, there is, once again, the choice to allow any sexual feelings to quietly fade away or to touch yourself. But remember, just because the genitals are included in the massage doesn't mean there's any expectation for you to feel highly aroused or to orgasm.

WHEN YOUR GENITALS are being touched, notice if you become tense. Have you begun judging yourself or analyzing what's going on? Do you feel unsafe? Do you feel embarrassed?

These feelings may disappear on the second massage, as you become more comfortable with the situation. If not, take some time to understand why you're reacting this way.

Perhaps you have negative feelings about your genitals. Unfortunately, some women do. In chapter 13 I talked about the need to feel comfortable with your vulva and clitoris. If you haven't done the Personal Change Program, and you're finding Step 3 of the Couple Change Program uncomfortable, I suggest you turn back to the previous chapter and work through Step 1 of the Personal Change Program.

If you're comfortable with your genitals, yet still feel tense during Step 3, you could be making a connection between what's happening during the massage and something that happened in the past that was negative or uncomfortable for you.

If this is so, take some time to look for something reassuring and positive to say to yourself. Try the examples I've given below:

---

- I don't have to do anything except this massage.
- I don't have to worry about something bad happening; this is a time for me to relax and enjoy myself.
- I'm safe and I don't have to be anxious about anything.

---

If these examples don't fit your situation, find one that does. Say it to yourself whenever you start to get tense. Remember to breathe deeply.

Are you still having difficulty with Step 3 by the end of the three (or five) massages? Perhaps you're still feeling guilty about relaxing and enjoying yourself. Or could it be that you feel uncomfortable when focusing on yourself? If you've been used to putting your attention on the future (or past), the experience of staying in the moment, without any distracting thoughts, can be rather scary. In this situation, emotions often seem stronger and more powerful.

There are many reasons for finding Step 3 difficult. See if you can identify what lies behind your own reactions. Talk to your partner. He or she may have some suggestions that will be helpful.

The exercise below may help you to sort out your thoughts.

## understanding my reactions
### finish these sentences:

1. If I were to let myself fully enjoy the exercise, I imagine I would think/feel/do _____

2. If I were to let myself fully enjoy the exercise, I imagine my partner would think/feel/do _____

_____

3. My fear about doing Step 3 is _____

_____

4. When I'm doing the exercise, I don't seem to be getting

_____

5. I could enjoy the exercise more fully if _____

_____

If necessary, go back to chapter 7 and remind yourself of the causes of your orgasm difficulties. This may alert you to the source of your difficulties at this stage of the Program.

Now try the exercise again, a couple of times, and see if your understanding of the problem has helped. If you feel yourself becoming uncomfortable once more, tell your partner. Try to work out what happened just before this uneasy feeling occurred. Was it something you thought about? Was it something your partner did? Remember to change any negative thoughts into positive ones. Then, if possible, continue with the exercise.

If you feel things are improving, repeat Step 3 another three times. And *another* three times, if you want to. There's no time limit and no rush to move on. Keep going until you feel ready to move to the next step.

If you truly feel stuck, see a psychologist or experienced therapist to help you understand the problem.

## STEP 4: building the pleasure

In this step carry out the massage just as you did in Step 3. However, at the end, your partner should return to touching your genitals, especially around the clitoris glans/hood and shaft, for another ten to fifteen minutes. You can also include touching inside the vagina. If the extra time is a problem, cut down the massage to twenty minutes, so you can add this new exercise. While stroking your genitals, your partner should also caress the rest of your body from time to time. You may also kiss (and have fun!). Of course, when it's your partner's turn, the same thing will happen in reverse.

Because extra attention is given in this exercise to your clitoris, you'll probably feel your sexual pleasure becoming stronger. The aim of this exercise is for you to *allow* this to happen. Learn to let your sexual feelings build stronger, but do not worry about feeling an orgasm. Let me repeat that. *Do not worry about feeling an orgasm.*

If you find an orgasm just seems to happen, that's fine. At this stage, however, orgasm isn't the aim. It's more important to learn how to let your sexual feelings grow stronger and stronger *while staying relaxed.* Try to allow them to become stronger than you've ever felt before.

At the same time, don't forget that sexual feelings sometimes dip into the valleys and settle onto plateaus. It's not always full steam ahead up the arousal hill. Accept these changes as natural, and you'll continue to build your arousal. Worry that you're "failing," "not going anywhere," "losing it," or _____ (fill in the gap with your favorite negative saying), and you *know* what will happen: your feelings will disappear.

Don't try to force your sexual pleasure to build. If you remember, the harder you try to have an orgasm, the more difficult it will be to feel one. On the other hand, the more you relax, imagine the warm syrup flowing through your body and take an *I'm-just-going-to-enjoy-what's-happening* attitude, the greater your chances of reaching higher levels of arousal.

It's very important, at this stage, to feel comfortable enough to tell your partner how you want to be touched.

**You may be more aroused than usual, and the kind of touch you need may change.**

*Show* your partner how you want to be touched. Put your hand over his or her hand and guide the touch. Talk about what you like. You may need to do this each time you do Step 4, if the kind of touch you want changes from one massage to the next. Don't forget to remind your partner of all the areas that can give you a turn-on, especially those that are under the skin (the branches of the clitoris, the shaft of the clitoris, the vagina, the G-spot).

Tighten your pelvic muscles from time to time. Squeeze as if you're pulling your vagina up into your stomach. This may give you a little rush of sexual pleasure.

If you feel a bit awkward when your partner starts to touch you, try sitting in front of him or her with your back pressed into your partner's stomach. You'll feel close and less exposed. Guide your partner's hand over your vulva and clitoris. It may not be as easy to have your vagina touched, but starting in this position can help you feel more relaxed. Later, you can return to lying down.

If you'd like to explore your G-spot or swelling of the urethral sponge, wait until you've been doing the exercise for some time; then get your partner to place his or her fingers inside your vagina and stroke firmly. Go back to the illustrations in chapter 3 if you need to refresh your memory.

Don't worry if it's hard to feel your G-spot. You may need to be *more* aroused for it to be felt, or you may not be very sensitive in this area. And, don't forget, if you're wearing a diaphragm for contraception, this can make it difficult to feel. Oh, and don't worry if you feel the need to urinate or wee when your G-spot is first touched. This is perfectly normal and will only last a few moments.

At the end of ten to fifteen minutes of genital touching, finish the exercise. If you wish to continue by touching yourself, do so. Continue to stay relaxed and avoid pressuring yourself to have an orgasm.

(*I know, I know,* I'm repeating myself—deliberately!) Remember, the focus is on enjoying your passion rather than orgasm.

If you've used a vibrator in the past and found this quite arousing, you may want to use it now to help build your sexual feelings. Try switching between fingers and vibrator, so that you don't get numb around the clitoris or fixed on the regular movement of the vibrator.

If you can do this exercise, move on to the next step in the Program.

℘

IF YOU'RE HAVING difficulties, take the time to work out why this might be so. Perhaps you've started expecting too much (you know what I mean).

---

> Well, I'm sure other women are probably having
> orgasms by now. It seems so ridiculous that I have
> to go through all this when others don't.

---

Oh dear! That's exactly what I mean about pressuring yourself. Just relax. All that negativity and pressure is not going to help. Why are you acting as if you're at the end of the Program—or should be? There are at least a couple more steps to go. Go back to enjoying yourself and let me guide you through them.

If you have a physical condition which leaves you unable to experience sensations in your vulva, clitoris, vagina, perineum, or anus, you may have found that another part of your body has become equally sensitive. If this is so, return to this area at the end of the massage. Focus on where you *are* sensitive, rather than where you are *not*.

If you have a spinal cord injury and wish to explore the possibility that you can experience orgasm through vaginal stimulation, then have your partner use a vibrator inside your vagina. You may find this is most arousing at a point deep inside the vagina near the cervix.

Some women have difficulty with Step 4 because they're afraid of becoming *too* passionate or too "out of control" with their sexual feelings.

You may have thought about this earlier after pinpointing the causes of your orgasm difficulties. Perhaps you identified a childhood message about keeping control of the sexual situation. Or perhaps you remembered an experience of being laughed at by an ignorant lover for the way you expressed yourself sexually. For some women, simply understanding the cause of their fear of letting go will be enough to help them complete Step 4.

However, for others, years of thinking and feeling negatively will have taught them to automatically tense up as soon as their arousal gets to a certain level. This can make Step 4 difficult to do. If this fits you, try the exercise again. This time, notice the point at which you start to switch off your sexual feelings. Take a few moments to see if you can trace the cause. Ask yourself:

- *What was I thinking or feeling just now that made me get upset as my sexual feelings became stronger?*
- *What terrible thing do I imagine would happen if I were to let my sexual feelings become stronger?*

Tell your partner your answers to these questions.

I think you know the next step. It's important to replace the negative thoughts with positive ones. If you're having trouble thinking of what to say, remind yourself of the Super-Positive Thoughts.

## super-positive thoughts

- I'm an adult. It's now okay for me to let my sexual feelings go.
- Being aroused and having orgasms is part of being human. It's alright for me to now enjoy my sexuality.
- I have a right to feel sexual passion.
- I can choose to let myself go whenever I feel ready.

When you feel ready, go back and repeat Step 4. Before you start, say the Super-Positive Thoughts to yourself. Say them again if you feel yourself trying to control the level of your sexual arousal.

Do this for as long as you feel the need. It doesn't matter whether you take another two weeks or two months.

If you feel really stuck, get help from a therapist who is able to work with inner fears and concerns.

## STEP 5: letting go

In this exercise you will repeat Step 4. The difference here in Step 5 is that there is no time restriction on how long your partner can touch your genitals at the end of the massage. However, you should touch for a *minimum* of fifteen minutes. See if you can allow yourself to enjoy being pleasured.

Let your sexual feelings continue to build. Focus only on your emotions and the sensations you feel in your body. **This is your time. Let yourself enjoy it!**

Don't forget to tighten and relax your pelvic muscles. Move your pelvis in a gentle rocking movement. Continue to breathe deeply, feeling the air glide into your stomach and right down to your clitoris.

As you gradually build the sexual pleasure, you may experience an orgasm. Don't worry if this happens on some occasions but not on others. Many women have this experience.

Having felt one orgasm, it's easy to build up your expectations of experiencing another one the next time you get turned on. Unfortunately, these expectations soon turn into pressure to "perform." Before long, you're trying too hard to make an orgasm happen—which, as you know very well, is the best way to make it *not* happen.

Accept the fact that the second orgasm may not occur immediately. Keep doing the exercise and, gradually, you'll learn how to relax and let it happen more regularly.

And another thing: don't worry if your orgasm seems to be over very quickly. This, too, is a common way of having an orgasm at first. Keep in mind that learning to build your arousal and orgasm is a skill and, like any skill, you need to be patient while practicing it. Keep in mind as well that there's no "correct" time that an orgasm should be felt for.

In Step 5, continue to tell your partner how you like to be touched. As you get more and more aroused, this might change, so don't assume he or she knows what you need. Talk. It's much easier than dealing with the feelings of frustration you'll get if you don't say anything.

Be prepared to tell your partner when you'd like to stop the exercise. You don't have to try for an orgasm each time. Learn to be aware of your mood, body tension, what you're feeling and thinking. These will tell you what's going on.

For example, you may be quite aroused, but feeling too tired to reach high levels of sexual arousal. On the other hand, you may have been feeling extremely turned on—until the baby cried and you started to worry.

When you feel your arousal go, tell your partner. You might want to finish doing the massage and come back to it later. Or you could do some sensual (nonsexual) massaging until you're in the mood again.

Use a vibrator if this helps, but continue to switch between fingers and vibrator.

If you catch yourself trying to stop the orgasm from happening, pause and take some time to think about why you're doing this. You could also ask your partner for his or her opinion. Sometimes a partner can see things that you can't.

If it would help, repeat the exercise until you feel comfortable with your feelings and reactions.

You could also move on to Step 6, where I discuss some other ways of getting turned on.

### STEP 6: exploring different ways

So far, you've been using *one* way of getting sexually aroused: touch by your partner's hand and fingers. However, many women find there are other ways that are more arousing. *Oral sex* is one. The movement of a partner's body against yours is another (*body contact*).

During oral sex, your partner's tongue and mouth are used to arouse you. The softness and wetness of these areas can be very stimulating for women. Many find this the easiest and most enjoyable way to orgasm.

In this step of the Program, you have a chance to explore your reactions to different kinds of touch. Let's start with **oral sex.**

First, I should mention that some women have learned to see oral sex in a negative light. They think it's unhealthy and believe their genitals give off an awful odor. The truth is that these thoughts are really fears, not facts. Provided you wash your genital and anus area well, and do not have any infections, there isn't any reason to worry.

If you have an infection such as thrush, get it treated and wait until it's completely cleared up. You should then be able to have oral sex. If you're infected with the herpes virus, you'll need to make sure there are no open sores before you do this step of the Program. If you're infected with HIV or hepatitis, check that there's no bleeding in the genital area and that your partner doesn't have a cut on his or her tongue or mouth. You should also find out whether your partner has any infection that could be passed on to you orally. Practice safe sex and check with your doctor if you have any worries.

You may find it helps to talk with your partner or a sexual therapist regarding your concerns about oral sex. However, there is absolutely no problem if you don't want to have sex this way. We all have our preferences, and no way is better than another.

For those of you who are happy to try oral sex, begin with the massage as you did in Step 5. When you get to the point of having your clitoris touched, have your partner do it with his or her fingers for a few minutes. When you feel ready, switch to tongue and mouth.

Just relax and enjoy the feelings you get. Do all the things I've mentioned before about letting go and floating along with the feelings.

Of course, you shouldn't forget to show your partner how you like to be touched. There's nothing that will turn you off more quickly than a tongue moving in the wrong way.

One last point about oral sex. Although many women find they orgasm best from oral sex, most men think of it as foreplay, rather than sex. So, just when she's getting nicely turned on, he switches to something else (usually intercourse), and her arousal is lost. Understandably, she is not happy! If you enjoy oral sex and find it arousing, then tell your partner you want to orgasm that way. You can still continue later with the kind of sex he likes.

✑

NOW, LET ME turn to using **body contact sex**. Follow the same instructions as for oral sex, beginning with the massage. When you get to the point of having your clitoris touched, your partner should stroke you for a few minutes with his or her fingers. Then you need to position yourself in such a way that your genitals are pressed against your partner's body (but there shouldn't be any penetration). Now, move your body in a manner that is arousing for you. It doesn't matter how you do this, as long as it's comfortable and easy for you to move. Continue for as long as you like. Try to allow yourself to become highly aroused and to orgasm.

### STEP 7 (OPTIONAL): orgasm with vaginal penetration

In chapters 6 and 10 I talked about women who believed they had a sexual problem if they couldn't orgasm during intercourse. Hopefully, this idea has disappeared from your thinking. You should now understand that intercourse without an orgasm is very common and that orgasms resulting from other ways of having sex are very enjoyable.

However, you may still wish to have the *option* of being able to orgasm during intercourse or when something such as a finger, vibrator, or dildo is placed inside your vagina.

As outlined in chapter 10, there are three things you can do to help you orgasm more easily in these situations: allow yourself to be highly aroused *before* your vagina is entered; *during* penetration keep your arousal high by stroking your clitoris or having your partner do it; and using intercourse positions that allow your clitoris to be stimulated directly. Let me show you how to include all these ideas.

Begin by having your partner give you a sensual massage to your whole body for twenty minutes. Follow this with the stroking of your clitoris (and if you enjoy it, your vagina and G-spot) for five to fifteen minutes. Switch over, so that your partner receives a similar massage. Then switch again, until you are both feeling quite aroused.

**If your partner is male**, get him to lie on his back. If his penis isn't erect, caress him until it is. He should also be touching your vulva, clitoris, vagina, G-spot, and other areas of your body while this happens.

Now sit across him with a leg each side of his hips. You should be facing each other. Because this position gives you more control over what you're doing, it is the best one for learning how to include orgasm during intercourse. It's also good for clitoris and G-spot stimulation. If you want to avoid pregnancy or infection, don't forget to use some form of contraception.

Now, when you feel quite aroused and wet, lower your vagina onto his penis and begin to move up and down. You may want to put some lubricant on his penis (or condom, if you're using one) to make sure you can move easily. If you feel your level of arousal drop, begin to touch your clitoris (or have your partner touch you) while continuing to enjoy intercourse. Try using your fingers, but a vibrator can also be used.

Another way of keeping your arousal high enough to orgasm is to lean forward to press your clitoris against your partner's body. Some women find this possible, others don't.

Please note, if your partner has an orgasm before you, there's nothing wrong with that. It's just human nature, so neither of you should treat it as a great tragedy! If his penis is erect enough to remain in this position, continue to touch yourself until you climax or wait for him to recover while enjoying some quiet (or sexy) time together.

If you want to delay his orgasm, either stop moving or let his penis slip out of your vagina and wait for his arousal to subside a little.

---

Mmm, but how do I work out whether
to stop or move?
What if I do the wrong thing?

---

The answer to both questions is that you and your partner need to talk about what's happening. Tell each other what you need in order to continue enjoying the sexy feelings. We're not talking about a lengthy conversation here—just a few words to say what you want. It will probably come out as rather sexy at the time.

When you feel comfortable doing this exercise, experiment with different intercourse positions. Some will allow your clitoris to be touched, others may make it difficult. Once you've learned which positions help you to orgasm, you can choose to use them at times when you want to orgasm during intercourse.

**If your partner is female**, you may want to be able to orgasm while a vibrator or dildo is being used.

Begin by having your partner massage you for twenty minutes and then stroke your clitoris for five to fifteen minutes. When you feel very aroused, allow your partner to place the vibrator or dildo in your vagina. When you feel your arousal drop, try using your fingers to keep yourself sexually excited. Your partner could also place her fingers or tongue on your clitoris. And, thirdly, she could take the vibrator or dildo from your vagina from time to time and use it on your clitoris, to increase your sexual pleasure.

Learning how to coordinate the touching of the clitoris and the vagina is a skill and can take time to learn, whether your partner is male or female. So be patient, and remember to have some fun along the way.

## when the program is no longer a program |

DURING THE COUPLE Change Program, many couples find that the Program stops being a "set of exercises" and becomes a "special time for ourselves." They feel closer, express sexual feelings with each other, enjoy touching physically, share a few laughs and intimate thoughts, and look forward to the time they have together.

Not surprisingly, after the Program has finished, many couples keep the massage as a part of their lovemaking. One couple I know decided to have a massage night once a month. They would begin by playing some romantic music while they ate dinner and had a glass of wine. Then they would begin a massage. Sometimes this would lead to sex. Sometimes it wouldn't. It didn't matter, because either outcome was seen as enjoyable.

Other couples have found that beginning sexual activity with twenty to thirty minutes of sensual massaging works well. It gives each a chance to unwind from the day and to feel "special."

Do you know, without the massaging I don't think I could get into a sexual mood. I'm so busy during the day that it's hard to switch over to feeling like a "lover." That twenty minutes of massage is just what I need.

And that's exactly how a lot of women feel. Make sure, however, that the massage doesn't lead to expectations that you *must* have an orgasm at the end of it. It's still okay to feel sensuous or sexually aroused without feeling you must orgasm.

# 15

# my final word

Dear reader, now you really *do* deserve a gold medal. To have stayed with me until the end is no mean feat! Just look at what I've asked you to do:

- look at your genitals *closely*
- face your fear of being too passionate
- confront being bored with your partner
- draw your vulva and clitoris
- be honest about your sexual needs
- find a flower which reminds you of your genitals
- admit when you feel embarrassed
- climb arousal hills, looking for a nice view
- talk about painful past experiences

Then there was . . .

- picture warm syrup flowing through your body
- change your sexual fantasies

- stop trying to please your partner so much
- learn to be less addicted to your vibrator
- stop having sex for a while
- do crazy quizzes
- find a spare hour, three times a week (hah ha!)
- let out your sexual passion in front of your partner

Not to mention . . .

- wade through my fury about the word *nymphomaniac*
- say positive statements over and over—and over again
- try oral sex
- *don't* have an orgasm
- accept masturbation
- put a lock on your bedroom door
- relax, relax, relax
- *and* open yourself up to change

Now do you believe me when I say you deserve a gold medal? In fact, if you've done a tenth of these amazing tasks, you deserve a pat on the back.

$\backsim$

ANY KIND OF personal change requires a degree of courage. This is particularly true in the area of sexuality. It doesn't take much courage to say, *I want to learn how to ride a bike, or I want to learn how to cook* (well, okay, maybe it does for those I-only-boil-water types). But saying, *I want to learn how to orgasm* is an act of bravery. So was buying this book. And so was reading it through. Congratulations!

$\backsim$

AND JUST IN case you thought that was the end, let me leave you with my most important message. **Never forget that:**

- I'm an adult. It's now okay for me to let my sexual feelings go.
- I can choose to let myself go whenever I feel ready.
- Being aroused and having orgasms is part of being human; it's alright for me to now enjoy my sexuality.

- Being aroused and having orgasms is part of who I can be. It's important for me to be me during sex.
- I have a right to feel sexual passion.
- I have a right to express my sexual needs.
- My sexual needs are as important as the sexual needs of others.
- Focusing on my sexual needs is the way to being more aroused; it doesn't make me selfish.
- It's now safe for me to find out about my sexual passion.

## Now that's thinking positively, isn't it?

---

Okay, okay, I'm getting the message.
So, is this really the end?

---

Definitely!

# notes

1   E.O. Laumann et al., *The Social Organization of Sexuality: Sexual Practices in the United States,* University of Chicago Press, Chicago, 1994, pp. 116–358.

2   J.R. Richters et al., "Sexual difficulties in a representative sample of adults," *Australian & New Zealand Journal of Public Health,* 27, 2003, pp. 164–170.

3   J.S. Simons and M.P. Carey, "Prevalence of sexual dysfunctions: Results from a decade of research," *Archives of Sexual Behavior,* 30(2), 2001, pp. 177–219.

4   H.E. O'Connell et al., "Anatomical relationship between urethra and clitoris," *The Journal of Urology,* 159, 1998, pp. 1892–1897.

5   H.E. O'Connell et al., p. 1894.

6   C.A. Darling, J.K. Davidson and C. Conway-Welch, "Female ejaculation: perceived origins, the Grafenberg spot/area, and sexual responsiveness," *Archives of Sexual Behavior,* 19(1), 1990, pp. 607–611.

7   B. Whipple and B.R. Komisaruk, "Brain (PET) responses to vaginal-cervical self-stimulation in women with complete spinal cord injury: preliminary findings," *Journal of Sex and Marital Therapy,* 28(1), 2002, pp. 79–86.

8   Laumann et al., p. 358.

9   D.F. Hurlbert, "The role of assertiveness in female sexuality: a comparative study between sexually assertive and sexually non-assertive women," *Journal of Sex and Marital Therapy,* 17(3), 1991, pp. 183–190.

10  Laumann, et al., p. 373.

11 T.L. Crenshaw and J.P. Goldberg, Sexual Pharmacology: drugs that affect sexual function, W.W. Norton & Co., New York, 1996, pp. 273–306; A.L. Montejo et al., "Incidence of sexual dysfunction associated with antidepressant agents: a prospective multi-center study of 1,022 outpatients. Working group for the study of psychotropic-related sexual dysfunction," *Journal of Clinical Psychiatry*, 62(3), 2001, pp. 10–21.

12 Laumann, et al., p. 358.

13 S.S. Janus and C.L. Janus, *The Janus Report on Sexual Behavior*, John Wiley & Sons, New York, 1993, p. 86.

14 Laumann et al., p. 358.

15 J.G. Modell, and C.R. Katholi, "Effect of bupropion-SR on orgasmic dysfunction in non-depressed subjects: a pilot study," *Journal of Sex and Marital Therapy*, 23(3), 2000, pp. 231–240.

16 T.Y. Ito, A.S. Trant and M.L. Polan, "A double-blind placebo-controlled study of ArginMax, a nutritional supplement for enhancement of female sexual function," *Journal of Sex and Marital Therapy*, 27(5), 2001, pp. 541–549.

17 Laumann et al., p. 85.

# index